Concepts of Pharmacy Practice

Concepts of Pharmacy Practice

Dr. Rajesh Bhaskar Nawale
M. Pharm, Ph.D.
Associate Professor,
Govt. College of Pharmacy,
Ratnagiri, Maharashtra.

Dr. Prashant Keshorao Puranik
M. Pharm, Ph.D.
Professor,
Department of Pharmaceutical Sciences,
Rashtra Sant Tukadoji Maharaj,
Nagpur University,
Nagpur.

Dr. Somashekhar S. Khadabadi
M. Pharm, Ph.D. FIC, LLB
Principal,
Govt. College of Pharmacy,
Aurangabad, Maharashtra

PharmaMed Press
An imprint of Pharma Book Syndicate
A unit of BSP Books Pvt. Ltd.
4-4-309/316, Giriraj Lane,
Sultan Bazar, Hyderabad - 500 095.

Published by

PharmaMed Press

An imprint of Pharma Book Syndicate

A Unit of BSP Books Pvt. Ltd.

4-4-316, Giriraj Lane, Sultan Bazar, Hyderabad - 500 095.

Phone: 040-23445605, 23445688; Fax: 91+40-23445611

E-mail: info@pharmamedpress.com

ISBN: 978-93-85433-91-7 (HB)

Dedicated to,

All fellow Professionals, our teachers and family members

Who encourage and stood with us.

Foreword

Introduction of post graduate course in Hospital Pharmacy at Delhi University in 1982 has started the revolution of Pharmacy Practice in India. Later in 1992, Govt. Medical College, Trivandrum started independent Pharmacy Practice Department. At around 1997 post graduate course in Pharmacy Practice was started by leading pharmacy colleges in the region of South India like JSS College of Pharmacy, Ooty, Al-Ameen College of Pharmacy, Bangalore.

Pharmacy Council of India (PCI), New Delhi, implemented Education Regulation (ER) 1991 with introduction of hospital, clinical and community pharmacy as main subjects. Outcome of this has changed the scenario of pharmacy education. The job of pharmacy professionals has crossed the boundaries from dispensing and compounding to the counselor and advisor to patient and physician.

In 2008 with the introduction of Pharm. D, a six years integrated course in India, the role of pharmacists in field of pharmacy practice is revolutionized. I am happy to learn that Govt. of Maharashtra has taken active initiative and started Pharm. D course first time in Government institute at Aurangabad and Amravati. In near future the pharmacy practice in India is going to be main stream profession for pharmacy students.

The authors of this book are actively involved in Govt. College of Pharmacy, Aurangabad for development of Pharm. D course and Pharmacy Practice. The experience, enthusiasm, devotion of these staff is outcome of this book. Authors have made every attempt to share their experience and expertise through this book. The book will defiantly quench the thirst of budding Pharmacy Practice students and professionals.

B. Suresh
President,
Pharmacy Council of India,
New Delhi.

Preface

Community pharmacist and hospital pharmacist has many opportunities for engaging new way of working. For the community and hospital pharmacist this new challenge is exciting as well as daunting. Exciting because pharmacist has many opportunities to do something new for society and apply his skill and contribute in health care profession; daunting because for the current pharmacist, this might be new territory. A motto behind writing this book is to make pharmacist aware for their role and responsibilities in health care profession. We have tried our best to make aware the pharmacist how they can use their skill, knowledge and attitude for better health care system.

The contribution of pharmacist in western countries like USA and UK is well known. The pharmacists over their play a vital role in the chain of health care system. Patients counseling, monitoring, advice to physician are some of the areas were pharmacist contributes a lot. However in Indian contest the scenarios is not that much admirable. The pharmacist first should know his role and responsibility in health care chain and should update himself to that standard so that he can contribute in it significantly. Pharmacy Council of India, New Delhi has introduced a new course named Pharm. D a one step ahead to this goal. Govt. of Maharashtra has taken a second step and started Pharm. D program in Govt. College of Pharmacy, Aurangabad and Amravati from academic year 2011-12.

One day community and hospital pharmacist will be a highly acceptable professional in health care management team. The overall aim of this book *"Concepts of Pharmacy Practice"* is to provide stimulus to encourage new way of working that will leads to increasing participation of pharmacist in health care chain. The journey towards this aim has already been started and by this book efforts are made to make this journey easier.

-Authors

Contents

CHAPTER 1

Communication Skills

Introduction

The process of communication develops from early age of child hood. New born baby communicate with mother *via* responding to her call. The process of communication is complex and involves various interactions with one person to other. In the process of communication information is transferred from sender to receiver. This information may be transferred using verbal language or non-verbal communication media. We all use various media of communication in one or other form. Communication may be with little thought or a serious consideration. The skill of communication has been developed from early age though interaction with each other. Pharmacists spend a large amount of his professional time for communication with patient, doctors and other health professionals. Many factors like language, social and cultural background, personality and many more factors affect communication. Effective communication is a key factor for a professional pharmacist. It will help him in communicating with fellow professionals and other colleagues.

Elements of Communication Skills

The elements of communication skills include Source, Message, Encoding, Channel, Receiver, Decoding, and Feedback.

The source is the process by which pharmacist formulates an idea to communicate to medical professional or patient. This process can be influenced by external stimuli such as charts, models, video films etc., or idea can come about by thinking about a particular subject.

The source idea is the basis for the communication and message is composed on this idea.

The message is what matter to be communicated to another party. It is based on the source idea, but the message is composed to meet the needs of the patient. For example, if the message is between pharmacist and physician then message will take different form than if the communication between pharmacist and patient.

Encoding is a way by which the message to be communicated is transmitted to receiver. The message is converted into a suitable form which will be understood by recipient after transmission. The encoding process is more important during patients counseling process. The medium of transmission will determine the form of the communication. For example, the message will take a different form if the communication will be spoken or written.

The channel is the medium of the communication. The channel must be able to transmit the message from sender to receiver without changing the content and exact meaning of the message. The channel can be a brief or detailed talk, piece of paper with drawing and words, a communication medium such as video film, telephonic message, oral message, sign and symbols or it can be a printed paper. The channel is the path of the communication from sender to receiver. An email can use the internet as a channel.

The receiver is the person who receives the communication. The patient or medical practitioner uses the channel to get the communication from the pharmacist. A receiver can be used a document or a file or in computer which depending on the above named channel for the communication.

Decoding is the process where the message is interpreted for its content. It also means the receiver thinks about the contents of the message and internalizes the message. This step of the process is where the receiver may compare the message to prior experiences.

Feedback is the final step in the communications process. This step conveys to the transmitter that the message is understood by the receiver. The receiver formats an appropriate reply to the first communication based on the channel and sends it to the transmitter of the original message.

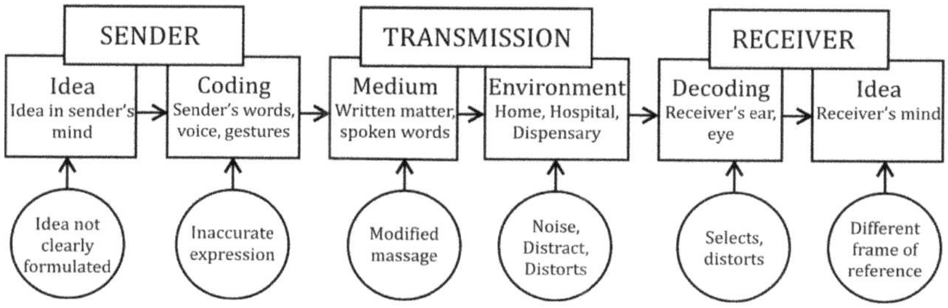

Guirdham (1995) developed a model to illustrate other possible sources of error at each stage of the communication process

Verbal Communication in Pharmacy

Verbal communication is a process in which a meaningful words or sounds are used as medium of communication. It involves speaking, writing, reading. Understanding the meaning of words is important in verbal communication. Change in tone, pitch, emphasis, language used alters the meaning of words. This aspect of communication is most ignored during communication skills. We communicate happiness, sadness, irritation during communication in our tone of speaking without realizing to listener and without altering appropriateness of words. There are two key components of verbal communications, 1. voice tone, language used and 2. content of message. Voice and tone add meaning to the words in the message.

Writing mode of communication lacks sensitivity. They produce exact meaning if written properly but do not indicate feeling of writer and dependent on interpretation by the reader. Different writing styles are also used for different purpose so that the exact message and meaning could be communicated. Some communications are quite formal like official communication letters from one office to other or emails. The tone of the letter is used in a particular manner to show the importance and severity of communication. Hence a written communication should be carefully drafted to avoid gaps in communications, and such communication should only be used for a particular type of recipient as per need.

Stages: In pharmacy practice communication lasts for few minutes. Time management is important during this communication process. The First stage of communication starts with

Introduction will become an important stage if pharmacist communicates with patient first time. This stage mostly repetitive during communication as pharmacy professional has to deal with different patients mostly. Stage of introduction will be of least important when communication deals with fellow or medical professionals as they may know each other in prior. The pharmacist should know language and other expected barriers of communications if any during introduction so as to have effective communication in future stages.

Opening is second stage. The topic to be covered should be introduced and briefly explained.

Business is third stage of communication. In this stage the main message and information is delivered and communicated and expected information is obtained from patient.

Reconnection is forth stage. Reconnection is preparation for ending the interaction. It will help pharmacist to make sure that patient/medical professional understand the details and relevance of the communication and obtain clarification.

Closure is the last stage. During closure non-verbal language also play important role. It gives indication for concluding of communication. Brief smile with handshake, bye signaling will conclude session. Closure should be concise.

Language: For the effective communication language used must be effective. Both parties must understand the used language comfortably. For example, a north Indian person whose knows language Hindi but know little English will communicate effectively in English with south Indian person whose primary language is Tamil, Telugu and Malayalam but know little English. Communication with common language but with different pronunciations and tones may prevent effective communication due to different meaning of words. Nature of communicator also works as a barrier for communication. Shy person speaks fewer words and admit that he/she do not understand many things.

Medicine and pharmacy are the professions which shares many common languages. English, Latin and Greek are some common languages used in both professions. Latin and Greek terminologies are different in various languages. These terminologies must be used with caution. It is most important that appropriate form of language with appropriate terminology must be used with a particular person during verbal communication. For example, heart attack is a common terminology used during communicating with patient where as myocardial infarction or myocardial ischemia will be appropriate word while talking with medical professionals. Use of such terminologies during communication with patients or during counseling should be avoided and common words should be preferred over terminologies in other languages.

Use of abbreviations in the prescriptions is for exclusion of patients from communication between medical and pharmacy professionals. Poor understanding of these terms may leads to dosing errors, change of overdose or in-adequate dosing during emergency situations. Pharmacy professional must comprehend these instructions and communicate to patients in his language so that patient could understand and carry out these instructions appropriately. Standard reference books provides listing of these terminologies to be used during oblique communications to be used by medical, pharmacy and other fellow professionals and will help to stay away from interpretational errors.

Nonverbal Communication in Pharmacy

When we meet someone first time, before the word is spoken we form a first impression about that person. The persons look, age, dressing, hostility, smell and many more give information. Unknowingly this information is sent by sensory organs to the brain and process large amount of information. With unconscious impressions and past experience, this information is compared and we make a quick judgment. Nonverbal communication involves the sending of messages without the use of words. This is the first impression and gives pharmacy professional much information about strategy of the further communication. 70 to 90% of entire communication spectrum is nonverbal. Further contact and verbal communication will add more information in first impression. Non verbal communication includes message conveying through body language and postures. A facial expression is important indicator of emotional state of a patient. Emotional reactions are associated with psychological status of the patient and may become a barrier for effective communication. Pharmacist must understand and recognize these barriers and take appropriate steps to overcome these barriers for effective communication. It is a continuous process and is the principle means by which feelings and attitudes are conveyed.

Facial expression, eye contact, touching, distance and personal space, gestures and movement, silence are some of the factors contributes and ways of the nonverbal communication. A man approaching you wearing a turban is Sikh. Well dressed person will have a good paying capacity. A patient with sad facial expression indicates he is in emotional stress. Approaching a person with smiling indicates happiness. These are assumptions about the personality we make from nonverbal communication. These assumptions are most of the time accurate and may be wrong some time and may become a barrier for effective communication.

Message conveying through body postures may help as signs of nonverbal communication enhancer or barriers. A person with closed arms and cross legs is known as closed body posture. Sifting feet, appearing restless and asking irrelevant questions are signs of in easy. This may prevent effective communication. Nonverbal signs such as looking else were, figure tapings are the indicators of non-attentions. These signals can be used to modify communication in order to grasp the attention of the listener. In this case appropriate action will be needed like temporary changing topic, offering a glass of water, asking questions regarding restlessness or their problem will grasp the attention.

Our face portrays wide range of emotions and reactions. Facial expressions can be read to understood or not clear about the communicated message. Eye contacts give different types of message. Glance of eye contact indicates involvement or confidence. Establishment of eye contact indicates interest in communication. Touching is an important type of nonverbal communication. It plays a significant role in older persons. Touch becomes effective media of communication in sensory impaired patients. Touching conveys warmth, caring, understanding, sympathy, compassion. More over touch is very individualized characteristic. Pharmacist should remember the comfort zone of patient during using it. The way people use distance or personal space is also a part of nonverbal communication. The distance between skin contacts up to 18 inch is close contact. Personal distance ranges from 18 inch to 4 feet, where two people are said to be in contact. Social distance is from 4 to 12 feet. Public distance is more than 12 feet. For the effective communication a personal or social distance may be used depending on the receiver. Movement and gestures are used to punctuate statement. The absence of words sometime is most effective way of communication. Words are always not necessary to convey message. Silence indicates hostility, anger, depression. It can express concern and caring. It can be used to defuse tension, offer time for consideration or interpretation.

Barriers of Communication

There are many reasons for failure of communication. The message to be conveyed, may not be conveyed or conveyed wrongly. The purpose for which the communication is done will not be served. The interpretation of message may be done in wrong sense, which may lead to adverse condition. Hence it is important that communicator should seek a feedback to check that the message is properly communicated and clearly understood or not. There exist many barriers of communications which may occur at any stage. Barrier may leads to distortion or wrong interpretation of the message. This will waste both time and money and put the patient or medical professional in confused or misunderstand condition. Effective communication should understand and overcome these barriers and conveying clear and to the point message. Common barriers of effective communication include:

- Use of over complicated and unfamiliar word
- Emotional status
- Lack of attention, interest, feeling irrelevance to receiver
- Difference of opinion, perception and view point
- Physical disability like hearing problem, speech difficulty
- Language difference and difficulty in understanding
- Prejudice mind leading to false assumption
- Cultural difference, non-assertive behavior
- Team diversity, task-preoccupation
- Anger or frustration, personal bias
- Lack of confidence, inappropriate priorities
- Organizational structure, distractions

- Tunnel vision, interruptions
- Rank differences

A skilled Pharmacist must take in account all these barriers to reduce their impacts on communication by understanding, continually checking and taking appropriate feedback.

Stage	Why error occurs
Sender: Idea	Ideas may not be clearly formulated before coding and transmission begins. For example, pharmacist wants to communicate to patient a precaution to be taken during taking medicines. He haven't thought about alternative ways forward the message written in complicated matter on box of medicine.
Sender: Coding	You don't have the right vocabulary to express your thoughts. You use overly complex language or jargon that the receiver cannot understand.
Transmission: Medium	The medium may modify the message. For example, if you communicate by telephone or in writing, the receiver cannot use your nonverbal signals to help interpret your message.
Transmission: Environment	The environment can distort the message. For example, noise on a telephone line could distort a message. Things happening around the sender or receiver (e.g., other people speaking, coming into the room, etc.) may distract them from the message.
Receiver: Decoding	Decoding may distort the message. The receiver may not hear the correct words, or may read written communications too quickly and misunderstand the message.
Receiver: Idea	The receiver's perceptions may distort the message. For example, their beliefs or mindset based on previous experience may create a barrier so that they don't listen to the message.

All these barriers can be classified in three basic classes as Physical, Semantic and Socio psychological. Physical factors refer to large number of physical barriers like noise, ill health, confusion, discomfort etc. Slightest noise like sneezing, dropping of object, banging of door or window, creaking of fan etc., creates disturbance, especially to listener, leading to loss of information. Thus during oral communication barriers like faulty seating arrangement, distance between two communicators, results in disturbed communication. In case of written communication illegible writing, poor photocopies also lead to disturbed or miscommunication.

Semantic barriers are pertaining to language varies from spoken words to written matter, chart or graphs. The receiver fails to get expected outcome of the communication if the words or expressions are too complicated or uncommon. The choice of words and language used by sender influences quality of communication. Semantic barrier occurs when sender and receiver interprets different meaning of the word and sentence communicated.

The socio-psychological barrier is outcome of attitude, emotions, status, source of communication, inattentiveness, poor retention, unsolicited communication, etc. Receiver responds to communication in very different way. Pharmacists used shortcuts during communication which results in incorporation of biasness into communication. Various shortcuts by pharmacist include stereotyping, projection of himself, use of monotonous words and language etc. Communication fails if their found a hasty judgment, refusal or ignorance to listen to the problem, fear of criticism, day dreaming, impatience, communication to two different individual simultaneously giving less attention to either, switching of discussion etc.

There are many ways by which all these communication barriers can be overcome and communication can be made effective, successful, and more acceptable. Easy practicable way of overcoming communication barriers can be used for this purpose. Physical barriers are relatively easy to spot and can be overcome by marking appropriate seating arrangement in quiet and confirmable environment. Audibility and visibility should be ensured visual and acoustic disturbances should be minimized. The environmental comfort should be provided. Linguistic barrier can be minimized using simple language which can be easily understood by the patient. A simple question during introduction will give an idea to pharmacist which language should be chosen for communication. Use of simple words, effective and simple charts, models, audio visual tools will also remove barriers of communication. Socio-psychological barriers are little difficult to tackle. It will be art of pharmacist that he will use different techniques for calling attention, motivating listener. Taking feedback at regular interval also lessen this barrier of communication.

Listening Skill

Verbalization is one side of effective communication. Other side is listening. The pharmacy practitioner should have a good listening skill. He should understand problems and difficulties of receiver. The question, queries, problem, formation given by receiver may not be important for communication but good listening will add in the rewards and better information for developing skills of effective communications. Listening skill is the act of hearing and responding to the content and to the feeling of what has being said. Words are often a cover up of what people feel. Most of us have acquired skill to use words. Pharmacist should learn to listen for the feelings that are behind those words. For example, in the statement *"I don't want to take this tablet"* the content is simply the information stated about the speaker not wanting medicine. The feeling could be that the speaker is not happy about something, dislikes the taste, effect, relief expected from medicine, or wishes to register a protest about something by not taking medicine.

Active listening is one of the effective tools of communication. Listening strategy is very useful to convey that you are interested in what being said, it shows that you understand that what the patient is saying, even when you do not agree for it. However listening is not always appropriate. Pharmacist may be busy some time and may not have time to listen. This may give negative impact of communication and patient may feel that pharmacist is not interested in communicating with him. This may become a communication barrier.

Effective listening is only accomplished through constant effort. Most people do not put efforts required to become a truly effective listener. We understood 50% of what we hear. There are many reasons for ineffective listening. One of the major reasons is poor listening habits. It is hard to listen critically or to listen for learning. You may require controlling the environment when listening is critical. To understand this we must understood the modes of listening, they are as follows:

- ***Competitive and combative listening:*** In this mode of communication receiver is more interested than speaker in putting his thought. When such listening occurs listener forces his point of view. Listener may pretend to pay attention while actually formulating what they need to say next. When this happened listener is involved in formulating their argument which results in confused communication.

- ***Passive or attentive listening:*** This type of listening occurs when listener is interested in listening and understanding the things. During this process good listener fails to take action.
- ***Active and reflective listening:*** This type of listening occurs when listener genuinely interested in the speakers message. Listener wants to know the thoughts and feelings of speaker. Listener always confirms that he understood everything before reaction to speaker's message. This type of listening is always very effective; most recommended and takes time to confirm that effective communication takes place.

Questioning Skill

The ability to ask the question and answer them is the questioning skill. Questioning is one of the most widely used social skill. It is central to learning process. Questioning is fundamental part of communication process between pharmacy professional and either medical professional or patient. Questioning should play a central role in communication process. Good questioning skill is asset for professional pharmacist. The use of questioning skill is important to investigate the depth of knowledge, understanding of the listener. The question asked may give idea about the use of language for communication, mental status of the listener etc. Because of this pharmacist must plan question carefully. The art of crafting good question is a key for effective communication process. This does not require any script writing but critical thinking, careful planning of the questions, which will guide him during process of communication.

Bloom classifies the questions. As per his taxonomy questions are classified in to six categories.

- ***Knowledge:*** The listener must recognize and recall the information, instructions given to him.
- ***Comprehension:*** Listener must think on lowest level so that without efforts he could reproduce the instructions given to him and without verbatim repetitions.
- ***Application:*** It requires that listener should do a simple mathematics like calculation of dose etc., with application of

the information he acquired from pharmacist during communication.

- ***Analysis:*** It requires that patient should perform a task like dose titration, body temperature measurement, blood glucose estimation etc., from the training taken.
- ***Synthesis:*** Requires that patient, his relatives should find out the solution depending on various situations. For example, Paracetamol tablet is to be given if fever is noticed, but the dose should not be repeated for more that 6 hourly.
- ***Evaluation:*** Listener, patient, his companion should make a decision based on the knowledge he acquired. This kind of questioner normally not used in medical professional because taking decision may be life threatening many times and let the decision be done by medical professional.

Types of questions: There are two types of questions - open and closed. Closed question is that which is direct and has a closed end. It is required that the answer will be a single word 'yes' or 'no'. Closed question give accurate information needed but it does not include feeling or emotions.

- Are you feeling uneasy?
- Do you feel good after taking medicine?
- Do you feel nausea after taking medicine?
- Are you taking your medicine regularly?
- Have you taken medicine today morning?
- Do you understand how to take this medicine?

Open questions are open ended and the respondent is allowed to give answer in his own way. Answering to open question provide more detailed information and no limit is set for it. Open question encourages elaborating and giving details of the information. The open questions build around words like what, how, describe etc. they allow to add feelings and emotions in answer. The answers to open question also give emotional status about patient. Pharmacist can also encourage the patient to give encourage and more information in answer. Some of the examples of open questions include:

- How you take your medicine?
- What are symptoms of your illness?

- Tell me schedule of your daily life?
- How you are feeling now?
- What doctor says about your disease?
- Did you discuss with doctor about your illness?

Using the combination of open and closed question allows the direction and focusing of ideas to obtain the desired information from patient. Pharmacist has to use this during communicating with patients. This technique is called as funneling technique. In this initially some open question will be asked to obtain basic information about patient like name, occupation, place, family background, nature and duration of disease etc., then asking closed question will provide specific information and clarity about disease. Afterwards the combination of open and closed questions can be used to obtain desired information.

Communication in Professional Practice

Communication with patients: Communication with patients is required for two purposes either for information gathering or for giving information. Information gathering is done during taking medical history. Information gathering is required to current medication treatment, for identification of suitable treatment, and for taking reliable medical history of patient. This information gathered will be used by medical practitioners for multiple purposes. Pharmacist records most accurate history of patients as compared to other health professionals. Pharmacist interviews the patient for recording the patient's medication history, experience during medication, emotional status of the patient and give suggestions and precautions during medication. Frequent interaction of pharmacist with patient provides an opportunity to strengthen pharmacist-patient professional relationship.

Communication with medical and health professionals: Pharmacist has to prove his credibility in pharmacy practice department to the medical practitioners if it is newly developed in the hospitals. To develop a good inter-personal relation, good communication skills and knowledge is most important component. Once these relationships were developed and accepted pharmacist has to prove his credibility. Pharmacist can be treated as a threat by medical professionals in their position and supremacy. His instructions and suggestions can be annoying during ward round by the medical professionals. Pharmacist should keep in mind the busy schedule and workload of doctors and should avoid unnecessary detail information and should only focus on patient related issue. The information provided should meet the standards and clarity. Short and clear statement should provide necessary information without creating any confusion. In order to fulfill all these requirements pharmacist must have strong listening skill, good and appropriate questioning power. Pharmacist should avoid all possible distractions to gather irrelevant and unnecessary information. Eye contact, body language, facial expression should be used as a tool for nonverbal communication. For the communication pharmacist may use various modes of communication. Telephone followed by follow-up document, verbal massaging, written communication in the form of document or presentation are some of the modes used for this type of communication.

References

A.J. Winfield, R.M.E. Richards (2004). Pharmaceutical Practice, 3rd edition, Churchill Livingstone.

Clara E. Hill, Larry Siegelman, Barbara R. Gronsky, Frank Sturniolo, Bruce R. Fretz (2001). Nonverbal Communication and Counseling Outcome; Helping skills, The empirical foundation; American Psychological Association, XVIII.

Dr. Arun K Behera, Prof. Bijay K Tripathy (2009). Barriers to Effective Communication and How to Overcome Them, Academe, Vol XIII, No. 1.

Fred C. Lunenburg (2010). Communication: The Process, Barriers, and Improving Effectiveness, Schooling , Vol. 1, No. 1.

G. Parthasarathi, Karin Nyfort-Hansen, Milap C Nahata (2004). A Text book of Clinical Pharmacy Practice, Essential Concepts and Skills, 1st edition, Orient Langman Private Limited.

G. Parthasarathi, Karin Nyfort-Hansen, Milap C Nahata (2012). A Textbook of Clinical Pharmacy Practice, Essential Concepts and Skills; 2nd edition; Universities Press (India) Private Limited.
http://www.immi.se/intercultural/

James Drogan (2009). Ethics, Critical Thinking, and Communications. www.pdnltd.com

Jens Allwood (2002). Intercultural communication; Business Ethics and Intercultural Communication; Issue 5.

K.G. Ravikumar, B.D. Miglani (2009). A Textbook of Pharmacy Practice, 1st edition, Career Publications.

Karron G. Lewis; Developing Questioning Skills; Improving Specific Teaching Techniques; Teachers and Students - Sourcebook; Center for Teaching Effectiveness, The University of Texas at Austin.

Mind tools on Active Listening; www.mindtools.com

Questioning Skills (2000). Westminster Institute of Education, Oxford Brooks University.

Remington (2005). The Science and Practice of Pharmacy, 21st edition, Lippincott Williams & Wilkins.

CHAPTER 2

Community Pharmacy

History and Definition

History: Pharmacy is part of life from humanity's earliest past. Excavations of (30,000 BC) support the fact that human gathers plants and herbs for therapeutic purpose. They use it by trial and error basis and depending on folk knowledge. Later in antiquity age the human learn the aspects of nature by farming shelter. Human became civilized. Clay tables are evident the beginning of rational use of medicine. At the middle age (400 AD) there was flourishing of Islamic civilization – Pharmacy. By the mid of 13th century practice of pharmacy was established first time in Europe. Arabic culture brings back the medical knowledge to Europe. The Universities start emerging in Europe like Paris (1150), Oxford (1167) and Salerno (1180). During 16th century Paracelsus who was a practitioner of pharmacy was originally head the chemistry. The apothecary Johann Hartmann (1968-1631) was first professor in chemistry at European University. This inclination for chemistry sustained during 17th and 18th century and at the beginning of 19th century it emerges as a separate profession. For around 300 years pharmacist contributes in the profession of chemistry of drug.

Pharmacy as a profession was recognized in 1700s to render services to the patients. Initially apothecaries were doing the jobs of pharmacist and take patients care. In the beginning of 1800s pharmacist acquire the role of medicinal chemist and its role as apothecary was left. Their attention was diverted from patient care to compounding of medicine and the apothecary was renamed as druggist. At early 1900s age old compounding was replaced by industrialization of pharmaceuticals. The pharmaceutical manufacturing replaced the manual compounding procedure at the pharmacy shop and the role of pharmacist remains restricted up to trading pharmacist. In post independent era Pharmacy Council of India was constituted under section 3 of Pharmacy Act for the regulation of education and regulation of pharmacy practice in India. In today's circumstance around 92% pharmacists are drug traders.

Now a day's India is country with house of many high profile diseases like diabetes, blood pressure, angina etc. The drug related problems are due to development of resistance, duplication in medicine, overdosing, under dosing, drug interactions, inadequate information to the patient, inappropriate dosing etc. The medical practitioners are becoming busy, and due to heavy loads of patients, they have limited time to focus on these issues. Doctors consultation is limited now to the prescription writing and no information about prescribed drug, dosing regimen and pattern is given to the patient. Community Pharmacy is the information provider in these issues. Again now a day's pharmacy is taking role of apothecaries. Community pharmacy has become information center for patient and pharmacist as an information provider. Now it is becoming a vital link between patient and doctor. Newly graduate pharmacist act as a responsible for maintaining all patients track and record, they do the job of patients counseling effectively and provide information regarding medication, diet and daily lifestyle. This will help the patient to save the time, energy and also the money because pharmacists may charge nominal amount for his services but at the same time saving huge amount and multiple administration of drugs which may lead to various side effects etc.

Definition: A group of people sharing common interest, living in a place and enjoying common privilege are known as community. Community pharmacy is the service rendered by the pharmacist to the community people in the benefit of their health care. Pharmacist caters the needs of society specially patients for their need of medicine. Pharmacist work with health care group and provide its services and handle the prescription related matters including medication, dosage regimes, cautions to be taken etc. Community pharmacy is operational area of pharmacy practice. It is many time more useful than Hospital and Clinical Pharmacy services. Pharmacist along with community pharmacy can also establish drug information center, poison information center, patient counseling center etc. In the Indian context community pharmacy means retail pharmacy store or a druggist and chemist shop where a prescription and nonprescription drug, health products trading is done. Also the counseling regarding what precautions are to be taken for that disease for example, diabetes keep the foot dry and clean do not work more time in wet area or keeping foot dry by wiping etc.

In the majority of pharmacies, the prescribed dosage forms are dispensed which are manufactured by various manufacturers who has Food and Drug Administration (FDA) approved manufacturing facilities. The dosage form meets the need of patient and manufactures under strict quality control and under good manufacturing practices which are recognized by FDA. Unique need of some patients for customized dosage form of medicine was fulfilled by community pharmacist. Patient may require a comparatively low dose (pediatric and geriatric patient) or high dose (adult with more than average weight and body surface area). Some patients may require a dosage form free from particular pharmaceutical aids like preservative, flavor etc., for all this compounding and dispensing of medicine is the main service render by pharmacist. Nowadays community pharmacists are paying their attention towards services to the patients. The increased need of health care also increases demand of pharmacy professionals. The following chart gives bird eye view of available pharmacies in various countries. The number of pharmacists required in the country depends on the health status of that country. Averagely around 6 pharmacists are present for 10,000 population word wide against the required number 1 for every 100 as per WHO.

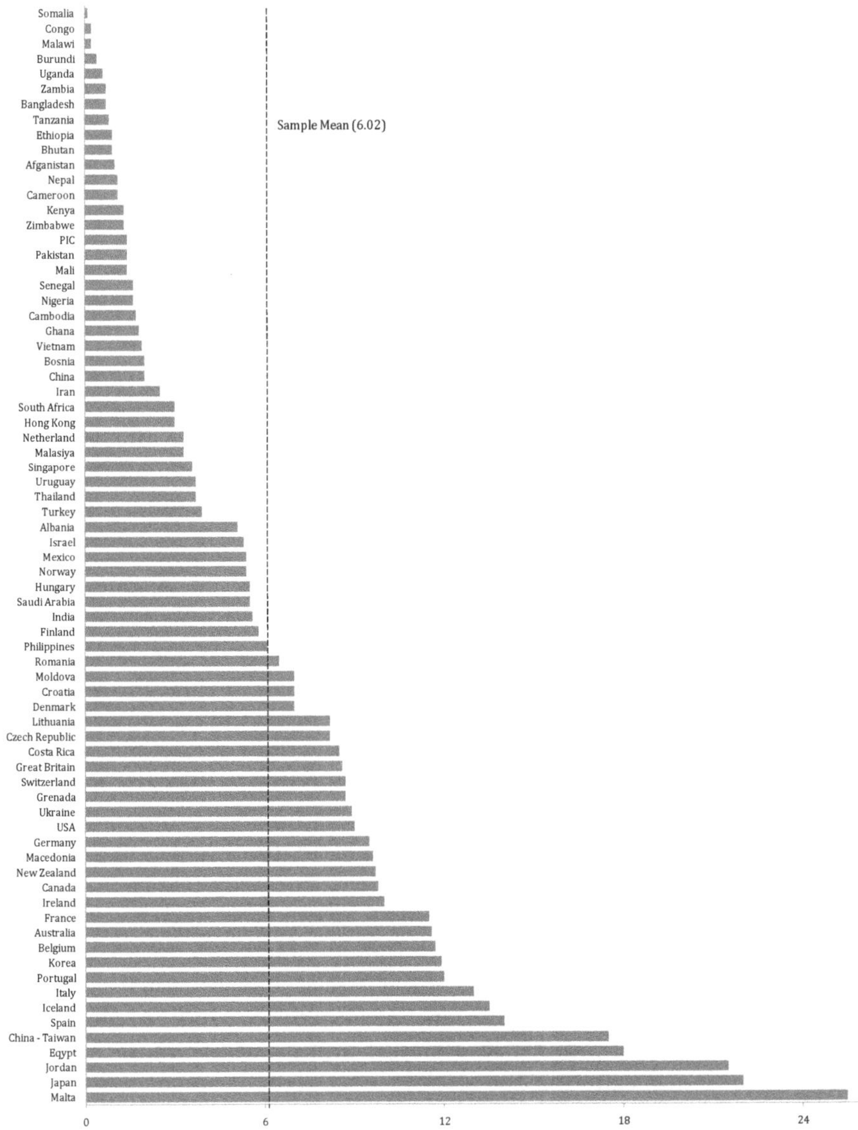

Density of Pharmacists per 10,000 population (Sample mean 6.02): Reproduced from 2012 FIP Global Pharmacy, Workforce report (available at www.fip.org)

Role, Responsibilities and Activities

A Community pharmacy is the place where pharmacist gets opportunity to have a social contact with community to reduce preventable drug-related morbidity and mortality. A community pharmacist is responsible for controlling, dispensing and distributing medicine in his shop. Pharmacist work as per legal and ethical guidelines provided by various authorities like Pharmacy Council of India, New Delhi to ensure the 'correct and safe supply' of medicinal products to the general public. They play a vital role in maintaining and improving people's health by providing counseling, advice and information as well as supplying prescription and non prescription medicines. Community pharmacists also provide over-the-counter (OTC) medical products and guide the patients for their effective use. Pharmacists can also provide non-specialist health check, facilities such as blood pressure monitoring and diabetes screening, and run a stop smoking clinics etc.

In India community pharmacy is considered as a one of the emergency service. It is the unique place of hybrid professionalism and business. Pharmacist gets unique opportunity to handle the matters related to distribution of drug, patient's advice regarding dosage regiment of drug etc. It's a point of contact between drug user (may be patient) and usages of drug for their beneficial effects, rational usage, minimum drug toxicity, maximum efficacy and cost effectiveness. Pharmacist is the principal source of information for the patients when doctors are too busy in their role and cannot devote sufficient time for individual patient for drug use as such they have little knowledge about the drug chemistry and biochemical pathways of drug which is most important factor to be considered and only pharmacist know this. Pharmacist has to work with full integrity with all the members of medical and health care professionals. Sharing of his knowledge and advice to patients make this profession a valuable for society and gives a social respect for him. As a team member of health care system or as a professional he is accountable to the patients for services provided. By his professional attitude pharmacist can become a vital member of health care system. Pharmacist represents third largest professional in healthcare system worldwide, but they are underestimated and underutilized in most of the developed countries including India. Community pharmacists are around 55% of all working pharmacists all over India. In European countries community pharmacists contributed for 60%, hospital pharmacists are around 30% and rest of 10% are working in different sectors like as manufacturing pharmacists, academics and other. In India over 90% populations are visiting community pharmacy at least once in a year. Pharmacist is proposed as a high priority and dedicated resource for public health with community pharmacy and expected to play a great role. Community pharmacists are at prime role in combating health issues and identifying risk factors for diseases.

Now a day's role of professional pharmacist has changed from traditional role as dispensing pharmacist, to sale of medicines or pharmacy trades to member of health care team. He now assists the public to get best possible results from medicaments by patient's education, counseling and patient's monitoring. Due to rise in world population it was realized that medical and health professionals are not sufficient to cater the overall need of health status. There is equal requirement of participation of pharmacist as a health professionals and Pharmacist are effectively doing it. Community pharmacy plays their attentive role towards patient's health, his environment, his status for wellness and counseling. The matters related to health diseases, nutrition, habits, addiction and drug abuse are also handled effectively by pharmacist. The competency standards for pharmacists in Australia were described eight functional areas covering a broad area of professional responsibilities.

1. Practice pharmacy in a professional and ethical manner
2. Manage work issues and interpersonal relationships in pharmacy practice
3. Promote and contribute to the quality use of medicines
4. Dispense medicines
5. Prepare pharmaceutical products
6. Provide primary health care
7. Provide medicines and health information and education
8. Apply organizational skills in the practice of pharmacy

Pharmacists working as a community pharmacist in pharmacies provide information about drugs sold without a prescription. Before suggesting a drug, pharmacists ask patient/customers about their symptoms and current medicines they are taking if any. He monitors patient's drug use and make sure that they do not take drugs that have harmful interactions. Pharmacists also perform administrative tasks like patient's record keeping and inventory on a computer. They analyze records to look at trends in drug use or possible excessive use. To summarize the community pharmacist performs following tasks in his job carrier:

- Review prescriptions for accuracy before dispensing.
- Provide guideline and information to patients about dosage, side effects, and drug interactions.
- Analyze prescription and trends in it to prevent excess usage and harmful drug interactions.
- Procure drugs and other medical devices as per requirement.
- Maintain procedures for quality, security and standards of the drugs.
- Maintain records of pharmacy inventory and patient profiles.
- Review and monitor drug therapies for hospital patients.
- Provide services to help patients manage special health conditions.
- Answer queries, questions and make recommendations to customers about over-the-counter (OTC) drugs.
- Advices hospital medical staff for selection and effects of drugs.
- Provide health promotion and prevention of diseases, activities.
- Provide training to pharmacy students.
- Refer patients to appropriate health care workers or physicians.
- Record information for patients and other health care professionals.
- Dispense drugs prescribed by doctors and health care professionals.

In addition to this main stream roles and responsibilities of community pharmacists may also get involved in various activities. In total these activities can be summarized as:

- Pharmacist will communicate health related information to patient in his language. He will counsel the patient regarding use of OTC and prescribed medicine. He records drug related problem, dosage regimen, proper method of drug administration, history, immunization schedule, refereeing patient to appropriate health professional/doctor.

- The community pharmacist may involve in area of Pharmacoepidemiology. It is the area where post marketing surveillance phase of clinical trial is done. Pharmacist records safety and adverse effects if any reported by the patient.
- Community pharmacist may also involve in counseling and advice for using family planning devices. He may also guide and make available the appropriate device as per the need.
- Community pharmacist may also involve in prevention of communicable diseases. He may involve in community campaigns and counsel the epidemic peoples. The spreading of diseases like AIDS, Hepatitis, Cholera, Gastro-enteritis, Plague, STDs, Leprosy and Tuberculosis can be controlled with the help of community pharmacist.
- Community pharmacist *via* his skills and active counseling can encourage the patient for progression of diseases, risk of overdosing etc. Managing blood pressure prevents chance of heart stroke. Blood pressure can be managed by regular checkup, appropriate medication, daily exercise and modification in eating habits. Similarly possible complications of diabetes mellitus like neuropathy, retinopathy, and glaucoma can be minimized by blood glucose monitoring and control.
- Community pharmacist can also involve in patient's health education using pamphlets, bulletins radio displays etc.
- Community pharmacist can provide counseling to pregnant woman about herself and child health/malnutrition, diet and hygiene management during pregnancy, possible sub nutritional diseases/pernicious anemia/iron and calcium deficiency and its impact on child growth. He can also educate parents regarding immunization schedule.
- Community pharmacist can also guide patient regarding nutritional values required according to diseases condition and importance of its requirement to early and effective cure of diseases.
- Community pharmacist educate community regarding environmental and seasonal diseases, diseases arise from

source like air, water and food born diseases, hazards and effects of pollution etc.

- Community pharmacist can also counsel the person involved in smoking, alcoholism, addiction, drug abuse etc. Hazards, drawback, side effects, social problem of these evils. He may refer these peoples to appropriate treatment, rehabilitation centers and health professionals.

Prescription

A prescription is a written order or written communication issued to the registered pharmacist by registered medical health professional (may be general practitioner, dentist, surgeon, veterinarian etc.) who is licensed to do so for providing medicine or other medical appliances for the patient. The prescription contains salient information regarding dispensing of medications. This order is usually given in the form of hand written, type written, readymade print with selection box or a computer printout. It may also involve verbal communication order from medical practitioner directly to pharmacist orally or telephonically. In some legal categories prescription must be written in the own handwriting of physician. Many of the time the prescription can only be read by his pharmacist, as the hand writing of doctors is very peculiar in some of the cases. Only the pharmacist can understand his hand writing for example, doctor has prescribed the vaginal suppositories but forgot to tell the patient how to use it and as a usual practice that patient took orally.

Prescription is a part of professional relationship between health professional and community pharmacist. It is professional responsibility of pharmacist to provide a quality medicine at reasonable cost that meets the demand of patient for cure of disorder. The pharmacist must be precise in dispensing of prescribed medicine and must give sufficient information to the patient regarding prescribed medicine. Pharmacist should assure that the instruction given by physician on the prescription is properly communicated to the patient and understood so that he will implement it in medication. Pharmacist must establish and maintain a trust of physician and patient. An integral part of this is maintaining confidentiality regarding the medicine taken by the patient and nature of illness. These are the personal matters of the patient and may give adverse reaction in social environment. In such cases maintaining confidentiality is prime responsibility of pharmacist. For example, if the patient is of HIV, STD diseases, tuberculosis etc.

Broadly there are two categories of medicines, the medicines which can be obtained by issue of prescription and those medicines which can be procured without prescription (OTC - Over the counter drugs). The drugs which are dispensed legally (other than OTC) requires prescription in approved format. The prescription is written by physician and given to patient to present it to pharmacist or it may be directly forwarded to pharmacist by a suitable route like telephonic, electronic or written format. The prescription order received by pharmacist verbally must be reduced in written matter.

The prescription are generally written by physician on printed form where the blank space is provided for writing the medicines, instructions and other required matter. The printed forms are called as blank prescriptions. The blank prescriptions are printed with name, address and other detail information of physician including registration number. This information clears the identity of prescriber. The prescription blanks are the printed form on which physician may write prescription when he visited pharmacy or when prescription was ordered verbally. These prescription blanks are printed with name and other details of physician. Specially printed prescription blanks is not a legal requirement of prescribing medicines, a blank paper can also be used as prescription blank with seal and signature of physician. Other than printed matter of blank prescription the prescription issued by the physician must contain at least following information. Certain information is mandatory for some class of the medicines.

- **Patient's information:** A full name of patient along with title like Mr., Miss., and Mrs. is must on the prescription for the identification purpose. Address of the patient is also mandatory field. Name and address should be written in legible handwriting. Incorrect spelling may create confusion for the patients bearing similarity in the name. Writing address helps pharmacist in dispensing the medicine if it is to be delivered to patient's home. If physician forget to write address, pharmacist must ask it to patient and note it down on prescription. Legal requirement make it compulsory to write name and address of patients for dispensing of some controlled substances. The address of patient is useful for monitoring and delivery of use of controlled substances. Also for cross reference and as history so that next time he can check the same.

Some prescription blanks also provide area for writing age, surface area, weight etc., of the patient. It becomes mandatory to write the age of patient if the prescription is issued to a pediatric patient below age of 12 years. This will also help pharmacist to check and calculate if needed the prescribed dose. Sometime the weight and body surface area is also required to calculate the appropriate dose.

- **Date:** This identifies when prescription was written. Prescription should always be dated when it is written and issued and also when it is received and dispensed by pharmacist. It is one of the important criteria for keeping the patients record and prescription record. The date of prescription is important when it is used for controlled substances. Legal requirement specifies that no prescription of controlled substances should be dispensed or renewed more than 6 months after the date of prescription.
- **Superscription (Symbol):** The R_x symbol is contraction of Latin verb *"recipe"* meaning *"you take"*. It is believed that the symbol originates from sign of Jupiter receive used by ancients to request of support in healing. Gradual distortion has lead to the symbol we used today. It is representation of prescription and pharmacist.
- **Inscription:** Inscription is the body or principal part of prescription. It mainly contains names, dosage and quantity of ingredients or medicaments. Now a day's prescriptions are written which contains already manufactured dosage by industrial process. The name of medication may be written as a trademark, trade name, proprietary name, generic name or individual formula. The pharmacist has to dispense the product as per trademark or suitable substitute having same ingredients. The generic substitution may be done to reduce the cost of medication. Some physicians write a specific line and allow or disallow such substitutions. Many times the information or type of dosage forms are written as abbreviations. Following table indicates various abbreviations used in prescriptions.

Short forms	Meaning	Short forms	Meaning
aa	of each	inj.	Injection
abd	Abdomen	IU	International Unit
ad	Up to	IP	Intra-peritonial
a.c.	Before meal	kg	Kilogram
a.d.	Right ear	L	Liter
ad lib.	Quantity as required	IV	Intravenous
admov	Apply	m, min.	Minimum
agit	Shake	mcg	Microgram
a.m.	Morning, before noon	meq	Milliequivalent
amp	Ampule	mOsm	Milliosmol
amt	Amount	ml	Milliliter
aq	Water	N.M.T.	Not more than
a.l., a.s.	Left ear	NS	Normal saline
a.u.	Both ears	oz	Ounce
BCP	Birth control pill	O_2	Oxygen
bis	Twice, two times	per	By or through
bid	Two times a day	p.c.	After meal
bol.	Large single quantity	p.o.	By mouth
BP	Blood pressure	p.m.	Afternoon
b.s.	Blood sugar	P	Pulse
BSA	Body surface area	q	Every
c.	With	qh	Every hour
Ca	Calcium	qd	Every day
CAD	Coronary artery disease	qs	Quantity sufficient
CHF	Congestive heart failure	RA	Rheumatic arthritis
cc, cf	With food	sig	Write a label
cc	Cubic centimeter	SC	Subcutaneous
cap	Capsule	SL	Sublingually
comp.	Compound	sol	Solution
CO_2	Carbon dioxide	s.o.s.	If needed
cr.	Cream	susp	Suspension
D5W	Dextrose 5% solution	syr	Syrup
dc, d/c	Discontinue	TB	Tuberculosis
dil.	Dilute	tab	Tablet

Table *Contd...*

Short forms	Meaning	Short forms	Meaning
disp.	Dispense	tbsp	Tablespoon
div.	Divide	tsp	Teaspoon
dm	Diabetes mellitus	tid	Three times a day
DW	Distilled water	T	Temperature
e.m.p.	As directed	top.	Topical
EtOH	Ethanol	T.P.N.	Total parenteral nutrient
fl., fld.	Fluid	u.d.	As directed
g, gm	Gram	U	Unit
gr	Grain	UA	Uric acid
H	Hypodermic	UTI	Urinary tract infection
HR	Heart rate	USP	United State Pharmacopoeia
h, hr	Hour	w	With
ID	Intra-dermal	w/o	Without
IM	Intra-muscular	wk	week

As per prescription, pharmacist must mix the medicine and ingredients, known as *Compounding*. A prescription must contain name of ingredients and quantity of each ingredient to be compounded. Name of medicine and ingredients are generally written as nonproprietary name of material. The quantity of ingredient to be taken must be written in metrics or apothecary system. Now a day's apothecary system as a measure of quantity is almost become nonexistent. The pharmacist has to calculate the exact quantity to be taken depending on the dosing frequency and duration of treatment. The abbreviations used in prescription should be clearly understood by the pharmacist, many times there might be misunderstanding between the abbreviations and may leads to incorrect dispensing or medication errors.

Now a day's most of the prescriptions are written with the name of medication which are readymade available and manufactured by pharmaceutical company at large scale. When the dispensing is to be done using such manufactured dosage forms the precaution should be taken with similarity in brand name. The pharmacist should take a due care to avoid confusion in such similarities in the name. The medicine to be dispensed may be available in more than one dosage forms like injection, tablet, capsule, solution etc. More over the amount of medicine in same dosage form may also vary. The dose of active medicament varies as per formulation. The prescription should contain abbreviation for dosage form and strength of medicament to avoid ambiguity in dispensing. Writing the dosage form is legal requirement of prescription. The strength of medicament should be written in prescription as variable strength product which is available in market. For example, a tablet with a strength of 2 mg or 5 mg of active medicament. The number of such dosage form, 10 tablets or 20 tablets depending on dosage regimen. Many times a regimen of dosage is available in a kit form, in such case the number of kit to be dispensed should be written in prescription for example, oral contraceptive kit, antimalarial kit. The duration of treatment should also be mentioned in prescription so that pharmacist can calculate the number of dosage form to be dispensed. For example, Instruction - tablet two times a day for one week, pharmacist will dispense 14 tablets. Tablet once in a day for 1 month, pharmacist will dispense 30 tablets.

- **Subscription:** Subscription is directions or instructions to pharmacist regarding compounding of medication. The procedure to be adopted and the labeling conditions etc. Due to diminished frequency of compounding, in the prescription the part of subscription is almost vanished from prescription because pharmacist has nothing to adopt any procedure for compounding the medications. Now a day's the subscription contains abbreviations designated to the dosage form (for example tab. for tablet, inj. For injection etc.) and the number of such dosage forms to be dispensed. For example, a term *fiat mistura* will be used to indicate prepare a mixture.
- **Signatura:** The signatura means instructions given to the patient regarding administration of the medicament. The word usually abbreviated as *Signa* or *Sig* meaning mark thou. The signatura is commonly written using abbreviations in English or Latin or combination of both. The list of abbreviations used in signatura is enlisted above. The instruction includes quantity/amount to be taken if intended for internal use, the frequency of administration or application, the route/mode of application or administration, the part of body to which

preparation is to be applied, special instruction if any such as 'shake well before use, for external use only' etc.

The pharmacist has to label the container of dosage form with appropriate instruction indicated in signatura. The directions given in the form of signatura has to be translated by the pharmacist and communicate to patients in his language because patient may be uncertain or confused about the terms used. Pharmacist may give directions and instruction in written form in the language patient can understand. Pharmacist has to use his communication skills to convey signatura to patient like the frequency of administration, best time for administration of dosage form, what to do if dose is missed. Pharmaceutical manufacturer many times includes a leaflet containing written instructions along with pictorial demonstration. The patient can learn how to operate special containers like inhaler using these leaflets. These leaflets are also known as patient's package inserts (PPI). The pharmacist also has to explain the expiry terms of the special medicaments like eye drop (for example, *use within one month after opening the container*), and about some antibiotic preparation which should be used within 7 to 10 days after the reconstitution. Physicians do not specify the expiry of medicine; they know that pharmacist provide this information to patient.

The confusing statement may be translated in simple form so that they can be easily understood by the patient. For example, a statement "Take two tablets twice daily" may be confusing for patients that, 2 tablets are to be taken in whole day or 2 tablets per administration and total 4 tablets must be taken. To avoid such confusion pharmacist may explain the same thing in sentence form like "Take 2 tablets in morning and 2 tablets at bedtime".

- **Renewal instructions:** Contains information about the number of times prescription be repeated. This information must be provided under renewal/refill information. Refilling of prescription is not allowed as per the National Health Service (UK). Two or more prescriptions may be provided instead of refilling the same prescription. If no information is provided in renewal it is understood that no refilling should be done. No refilling is permitted for controlled substances.

- **Name and Signature of Prescriber:** Finally prescription should bear name, seal and signature of prescriber along with highest degree and registration number. Signature on the prescription is legal requirement of prescription.

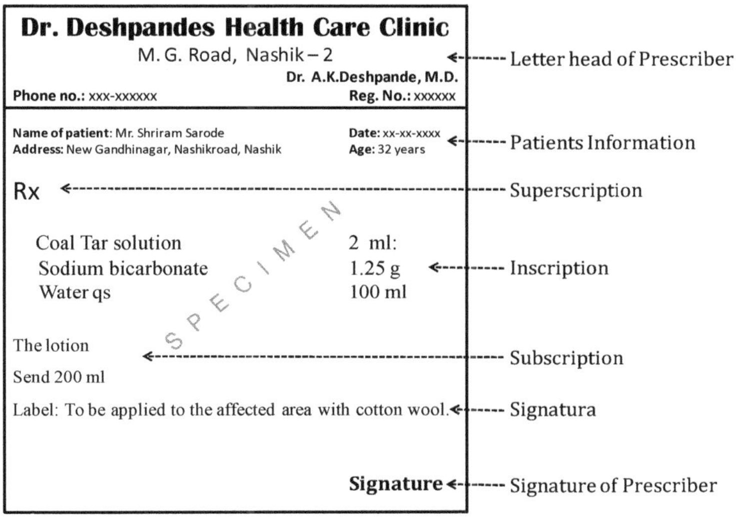

Specimen prescription for Schedule H drugs

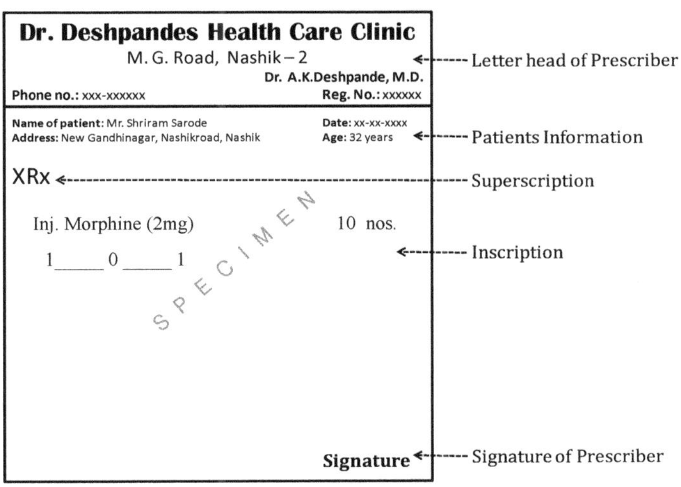

Specimen prescription for Schedule X drugs

e-prescription

Now a day's prescription is a vital part of health care system. The patient visited the physician; physician examines patient and give a piece of paper on which list of medication is written known as prescription. Poor handwriting, improper instructions on prescription, similarity in the name and strength of medicament, and other ambiguities leads to errors in prescriptions. Errors in prescription many times may be lethal to the health of patient. It is therefore recommended that prescription should be written electronically.

The electronic prescription (e-prescription) is a computerized physician order electronically transmitted to the pharmacist computer. In e-prescription, after the diagnosis of patient, physician will make entry in computer system regarding medication to be prescribed, dosage regimen, instructions to the pharmacist, the instructions to be given to the patients by pharmacist etc. Computer software may provide additional information regarding alternative drugs available, cost effective drugs etc. This e-prescription will be transmitted to the pharmacist's computer which is connected *via* LAN or internet to physician computer. The patient was given a unique identification number, which he will give to the pharmacist and collect the medicine from him. Patient will understand the instructions regarding medicine usage.

The traditional handwritten prescriptions from the doctors are more acquainted for the patient. Taking the prescription to pharmacy and getting it dispensed is routine procedure during treatment. In e-prescription computers technology and software are used. Everything works on an electronically secured system in standard format. e-prescription are ready with pharmacist before patient reaches to the pharmacy. There is tremendous reduction in number of unfilled prescription and it make easy to patient to have a properly filled prescription.

e-prescription increases safety, saves time, reduces medication errors, waiting time in pharmacy and cost of therapy by use of generic medicine instead of branded drugs. Physician and pharmacist have easy access to medication history, allergic conditions if any, ease to determine drug-drug or drug food interaction, ease in decision making and proper counseling to the patient. e-prescription cannot be a substitute for traditional prescribing when prescribing controlled substances where there is a legal requirement of suitable prescription (for example – prescription in triplicate when drugs like narcotics are to be prescribed). The physician, pharmacist and patient should not expect that there will be a complete absence of mistakes and errors in e-prescriptions. This is an advanced technique with many suggestions at different levels, history recording, physician's decision making during diagnosis, and prescribing medication, patient mental condition during conversation with physician, work load of pharmacist may play vital role during working on e-prescriptions. There may not be any information regarding new drugs and formulations coming in the market and other information like drug/food interaction there off. This requires regular update of software with recent information.

Review: At the time of dispensing, a prescription must be reviewed for various information like prescription number, date on which the prescription was dispensed, manufacturer's drug identification number or the brand name of the product dispensed, the quantity dispensed. A pharmacist must review prescriptions for completeness and appropriateness with respect to the drug, dosage, route and frequency of administration. He must review patient personal health information for potential drug interactions, allergies, therapeutic duplications and any other potential problems, patient's drug history and other personal health information, follow-up on suspected adverse drug reactions.

Errors: Errors and mistakes in medical care can occur anywhere in the health care system, at hospitals, doctor's offices, nursing homes, pharmacies, or patients' homes and in any part of the treatment process involving wrong medication, improper treatment, improper handling of prescription or incorrect or delayed test results etc. However errors in prescription handling can be minimized if proper care is taken. Medication errors can be reduced by replacement of sloppy hand writing with computerized prescription is effective way of reducing errors in prescriptions. Poor oral communication can be potential site of error. Enhanced communication skill and better interaction will help in reducing this error. Writing the prescription in full order in plain English rather than use of confusing short forms or abbreviations which leads to misinterpretation may also reduce the potential errors in the prescriptions. During writing the prescription on paper use of trailing zero, missing of decimal point may leads to 10 fold increases in dosing to the patient. Slight modification in pattern may reduce these errors. For example, writing 1 mg will always helpful instead of writing it as 1.0 mg. Missing or non-reading of decimal will leads to 10 fold increases in dose. Writing the word daily as an indication of dosing frequency will help a lot instead of writing it as qd which can be taken as qid meaning four times a day or qod meaning every other day.

Although the contribution of prescription errors that occurred in medication of patients is around 11 to 14%, it's a significant figure and cannot be overruled. An error in medication occurs mainly due to 5 reasons. Wrong drug, wrong dose, wrong route, wrong time and wrong patient. Prescription can be a common reason for all these five wrongs. Careful monitoring and pharmacists alertness may reduce the errors in prescriptions.

Handling of Prescription

The prescription handling is the first and the basic step involved in the community pharmacy and the pharmacist should be very good in handling the prescription. The prescription handling involves the following steps:

- Receiving prescription
- Checking prescription
- Preparing medication
- Medication dispensing
- Recording prescription
- Counseling
- Miscellaneous

Receiving prescription: It is desirable that patient should handover the prescription directly to the pharmacist. The prescription should be received in professional manner. The prescription should not be received with amazement or the shock on the face so that the patient should feel bad and think that there is something wrong in the prescription or he/she is suffering from some serious disease. The prescription should be received with good smiling face and any information obtained from prescribed drugs should not be disclosed unless and until it is the requirement of prescription or patients counseling.

Checking prescription: Once the prescription is received from patient, the prescription must be read and checked carefully and completely by the pharmacist before dispensing of the drug. There should not be any doubt about any ingredient and quantity of the prescription. In case of any mistake or doubt in the prescription reading to the spelling of the drug or their dose or any other problem, the pharmacist must refer it to prescriber who has prescribed the prescription. The pharmacist is not allowed to make any changes in the prescription without the order or notice of the prescriber. It's the clear responsibility of the pharmacist to check the legal requirement of prescription if any before dispensing the prescription. Pharmacist should check compatibility of medicine (especially newly prescribed drugs) with other drugs prescribed. Most of drug-drug or drug-food interaction will be identified by computer software. However information regarding newly introduced drugs may not be available in the computer software and pharmacist must be cautious during dispensing of these medicines.

Preparing medication (compounding): After reading and checking the prescription pharmacist should make a plan how to prepare the medicine. The medication to be dispensed should be prepared by pharmacist with lot of care. The pharmacist should use the correct weight and measures to dispense the drug. The pharmacist should not prepare a medication with the presumption or approximation. During compounding the prescription pharmacist should take in to account the physical and chemical compatibility of ingredients, the proper order of mixing ingredient, need of special adjuvant and special technique if any. The pharmacist should not dispense the substandard or adulterated or spurious drugs. The pharmacist should not also dispense the schedule G, H and X drugs without the prescription to anyone and should also not refill it without the prescription.

Medication dispensing: The dispensed drugs should be packed in the suitable packing material to avoid any mishandling or confusion during administration. The pharmacist should select the containers depending on type and quantity of medicament. Every dispensed prescription must be rechecked, the ingredient and amount must be verified by the pharmacist. Rechecking is very important when dosage forms are available in multi strength. The pharmacist should be personally present during dispensing.

Recording prescription: The record of the prescription dispensed should be kept in the pharmacy using computer. The Pharmacist should charge right price from the patient including the taxes, prescription handling charges etc. The pharmacist should not charge any hidden cost from the patient. The pharmacist must make a fair and adequate profit.

Counseling: The pharmacist should counsel the patient for few minutes while dispensing the drug. The pharmacist should tell the patient about the proper administration of drug and the proper dose and time of taking of the drug.

Miscellaneous: The pharmacist should at last verify the whole prescription before handing over the drugs to the patient.

Types of prescriptions

The prescription received by pharmacist may be of different types depending on prescriber. The prescriptions can be divided in following categories.

- Private prescriptions
- NHS (Nation Health Service) prescriptions
- Hospital prescriptions
  - Prescription for hospital inpatients
  - Prescription for hospital discharged patients
  - Prescription for hospital outpatients
- Legal prescription

Private prescriptions: The private prescription is given by family doctors, physician and veterinarian. This prescription is for medication of individual or veterinary use. These types of prescription are normally hand written by prescriber on notepad and has R_x symbol on it. The symbol R_x is generally used in private prescriptions. Dispensing of private prescription is entirely different from NHS prescription in several aspects. The patient pays a cost of dispensing to the pharmacist, which includes the cost of medication, container, professional service charges of pharmacist and taxes. The pharmacist keep record of dispensed prescription in his register and write a reference number of this register on label of container with stamp. During dispensing of controlled substances a copy of prescription should be retained for record by pharmacist and in other dispensing the prescription is handed over to patient.

NHS prescriptions: The NHS prescription is issued by medical professionals who have a contract with NHS and these prescriptions are only issued to NHS patients. Physician prescribes medicines and drugs from the list of NHS. The NHS prescription is issued in standard FP10 form. The form FP10 has different 9 subtypes depending on type of FP10 forms (e.g., printed form, printed pad, computer generated print etc.), prescriber (physician, dentist, nurse etc.), drug to be prescribed (e.g., NHS prescription form FP10 MDA and FP10 (HP) Ad. for methadone).

The NHS prescription has 3 parts at front side. The first part (A) of NHS prescription contains details of medicine and quantity of each medicine, instruction to the patients, signature of prescriber and date. The box at top also contains number of day's treatment which is helpful for pharmacist to calculate the quantity of medicine to be dispensed. The second part (B) of prescription gives details of patients which comprises of name, age and address. The third part (C) of prescription is endorsement by pharmacist. This consists of stamp of pharmacist, information about pack and quantity dispensed by pharmacist etc. The pharmacist has to endorse information during dispensing.

For NHS prescription patient do not pay to the pharmacist. The levy is charged on each prescription in respect of medicine dispensed. Pharmacist collects this levy on behalf of NHS. The payment for dispensing to pharmacist is paid by NHS on per month basis. After dispensing the copies prescriptions are sent to pricing authority of NHS and payment are made by these authorities.

Hospital prescriptions: Hospital prescription does not have standard format. The prescription has space for writing medicine and separate space for nursing staff for noting the details about administration of medicine. Hospital uses the prescription as an order for dispensing as well as record of administration. Different hospitals prepared different format depending on administration of drugs to the patients, like regular administration, one time administration or administration of drugs as and when required.

The prescription used for hospital inpatients comprises of space for writing the list of medication and space for recoding of details about administration. The prescriptions also contain details about patient's identification like name, address, age etc. Along with name of drug it also contains information regarding dose of drug, route of administration, frequency and time of administration. Depending on stay of patient in hospital prescription form may be vary in design. Short stay patient most of time requires one time administration of drugs like pre-anesthetic medication before surgical operation or it may require administration of drugs on regular basis like antibiotic regimen. One time administration drug and regular administration drugs are written in separate sections. Regular basis administration drug also contains drugs to be administered as and when required like post-operative administration of drugs like sedatives, laxative etc. In such condition each ward has a separate stock of drugs for administration of patient as and when required. This stock may be dispensed on the prescription of nursing staff of the ward. The administration of drug to the patient during his hospitalization is recorded on patient's record and cost is recurred from patient's medical bill.

The second type of prescription given in hospital is for dispensing of medicines which are to be taken by the patients with them during discharge from the hospital ward. The prescription form may be similar to that of outpatient or as a separate section in the prescription of inpatients. A bulk quantity of drugs for 1 or 2 weeks may be supplied to the patients during discharge and if necessary patient can obtain further drug requirement by the prescription of physician from pharmacy. The drugs which are supplied at the time of discharge will be filled in patient's medical record.

The third category of prescription is prescription given to the patients which are hospital outpatient. The prescription format will be only valid and available for that particular hospital use only. The details on the form include details of patient's identification like hospital registration number, name, address, age etc. The supply of medicine is policy decision. The quantity supplied may be for 1 or 2 weeks or quantity sufficient to meet the need till next appointment with physician. The record of dispensed medicine will be kept with patient's record in the hospital and copy in the pharmacy.

Legal prescription: A legal prescription is the prescription that fulfills all the criteria required for dispensing of the prescription. The legal prescription must contain all the information describes above. The information regarding prescriber contains its name, qualification, address, contact number and registration number. The information regarding patient includes name, address, age, sex date, weight etc. the part of the inscription must contain abbreviation regarding nature of dosage form, name of medication, its dose, quantity of medication to be dispensed etc. The part of subscription must contain all the relevant information regarding instruction to the pharmacist for dispensing of medication and instruction to be given to the patient regarding dosing regimen, precaution etc. To fulfill the final criteria prescription must contain a dated signature of prescriber, without which prescription will not be considered as a legal prescription.

The legal requirements for different types of prescription are different. A private prescription can be a single paper handwritten or computer generated fulfilling all the above stated criteria but a prescription for dispensing of controlled substances must be in triplicate, without which the prescription will not be treated as legal prescription.

Interpretation of Medication Order

The prescription is a medication order issued by physician to the pharmacist to dispense the drugs or appliances for use of patients; it also involves the instructions to the nursing staff for preparation of dosage form, dose to be administered and frequency of administration. The prescription issued by the physician may be hand written or computer generated. There might be use of abbreviations in the prescription writing. Computer generated prescriptions might not create much problem but hand written prescriptions containing use of confusing abbreviation may leads to misinterpretation and leads to errors in medications. After issue of prescription it was mainly interpreted at two places, first during dispensing at pharmacy and secondly at hospital during administration by nursing staff. Some time it will also be interpreted by patients for self-administrating prescriptions.

Interpretation of prescription during dispensing by the pharmacists plays important roll. Misinterpretation may leads to wrong calculation of dosage form, formulation and dispensing of product with over or under strength dosage form, use of drugs with confusing names, wrong counseling of patient due to misinterpretation of the instructions. Pharmacist should take due care to avoid these misinterpretations. After receiving the prescription it should be read and checked for its content, signatura and legal aspects. The content of prescription should be understood clearly for their identity and quantity to be taken for dispensing. Any ambiguity should not be overlooked and assumptions should not be made. Ambiguous names and quantity must be cleared from prescriber. Pharmacist may use his past experience, knowledge and information obtained from patient during introduction to check the correctness in inscription. The content of signatura must be clearly understood; the container should be labeled with signatura and communicated to the patient in his language. The interpretation of signatura plays important role for timely administration of drug. The pharmacist should first interpret the signatura clearly and properly and communicated to the patients. The effect of the medication depends on proper, timely, adequate administration of dose and patients counseling by the pharmacist has important role in it.

The second place where the interpretation of prescription plays important role is nursing staff in the hospital. The nursing staff has to understand the instruction given regarding drug administration. After reading the instruction they have to calculate and prepare exact dose for the patient. The patient to whom the drug is to be administered is identified because hospital ward may contain many patients with similarity in name, disease pattern and drugs to be administered. The route by which drug is to be administered must be understood and dosage administration is done. A proper record of drug administration is made in patients card and patient is monitored for desired effect and adverse effect any. The drug order to be remembered by the nursing staff include patients name, name of drug, dosage, route of administration, frequency, time and special instructions given (if any), date and time of order, signature and other details of prescriber. A precaution must be taken during interpretation that any part of order is missing or unclear, the order is incomplete and not fulfilling legal requirement, it has difficulty in interpretation and instruction cannot be understood. A word of clarification must be obtained from prescriber instead of improper interpretation of the medication order. The commonly found abbreviations and names of drugs leading to misinterpretation are listed below.

Abbreviation	Meaning	Misinterpretation
μg, mcg	microgram	Mg – milligram
BT	Bed time	BID – twice daily
cc	Cubic centimeter	u – unit

***Table** Contd...*

Abbreviation	Meaning	Misinterpretation
IJ	Injection	IV – Intravenous
IU	International unit	IV – Intravenous
IN	Intranasal	IV or IU
q.d.	Once daily	q.s. – quantity sufficient
SC	Subcutaneously	SL – sublingual
1.0 mg	1 mg	10 mg
.5 mg	0.5 mg (1/2 mg)	5 mg
ss	Sliding scale of insulin	Read as 55
Dp	Latin term Drachm	Symbol taken as 3

Drug name	Misinterpretation	Drug name	Misinterpretation
Albuterol	Atenolol	Hydralazine	Hydroxyzine
Chlorpromazine	Chlorpropamide	Lorazepam	Alprazolam
Cefoxitin	Cefotaxime	Methotrexate	Metolazone
Clonidine	Klonopin	Penicillin	Penicillamine
Digitoxin	Digoxin	Physostigmine	Pyridostigmin
Diphenylhydramine	Diphynhydrinate	Prednisolone	Prednisone
Doxirubicin	Daunorubicin	Quinidine	Clonidine
Dopamine	Dobutamine	Quinine	Quinidine
Enalapril	Anafranil	Ramapril	Enalapril
Folic acid	Folinic acid	Timolol	Atenolol, Tylenol
Glipizide	Glyburide	Vinblastine	Vincristine

Health Education

According to the WHO (1948), "Health is a state of complete physical, mental and social well-being and not merely an absence of disease or infirmity so that each citizen can live a socially and economically productive life". There are main three dimensions of health includes physical, mental, social status of individual. Beside this other dimensions includes Emotional, Vocational, Philosophical, Cultural, Socio-economical, Environmental, Political, Educational, Nutritional status. To understand the strength and need of community health assessment programs are undertaken. This provides baseline about health of community, ensures that decisions are based on authentic information; it helps to set the priority and information obtained can be used to guide policy development etc. Health care is the services render to the individual or his family by the health care services or professionals for promoting, maintaining, restoring the health. All health care systems has one common thing that the community for which healthcare is provided. The term medical care is the personal services provided by physician directly to the patient or individual. A healthcare system refers to a system developed for providing health care to the personals. Community health is a health status of members of community. Public health is the science and art of preventive disease, prolonging life span, promoting health, sanitation of environment, control of communicable diseases, education of individual for personal and community health and hygiene, nursing services for diagnosis, prevention and treatment etc.

Public health refers to health status of organized community, whereas community health is healthy status of members of community. Public health is a part of community health. The main objective of public health is to control the environments in which community persons are living, whereas community health take care of physical, mental, social status of the individual. In community health community practitioner is not needed, instead a community involvement and its participation is required. Pharmacist can keep pamphlet and brochures regarding various services free of cost at the pharmacy so that anybody who need can use them.

The International Pharmacy Federation (FIP) has provided guidelines for Good Pharmacy Practice (GPP) consisting of mission regarding providing medication and other health services and health education to the people and society. The concept of GPP mainly based on role of pharmacist in pharmaceutical care and health service providing including patient's care and health education. The primary objective of healthcare is to improve life quality of patient, which can be achieved by giving better health care facilities. Patient should be aware about the concept of healthcare and health education to avail these facilities in better sense.

Community pharmacist provides important services for all other health care providers and facilities to their community. They also served for inpatient and outpatient health organizations. Pharmacist also offer additional healthcare checkup facilities like blood pressure, blood glucose level, diabetes counseling, tobacco and alcohol cessation, cholesterol and osteoporosis management and immunization programs. Pharmacist can become a vital member of organization team of educational programs and workshops suitable for male and female participants, including teens, adults and parents. Single and multi-session workshops and presentations can be tailored to meet specific needs. In such programs various health education topic can be included like sexuality, puberty, pregnancy and healthy relationship, HIV and STD etc. They can also be educator for family planning service provider, parent-child communication and parental involvement, adolescent health and development.

Mass campaigns and development of new techniques are some tricks used for prevention and control of communicable diseases. Epidemic diseases like malaria, poliomyelitis, cholera, plague, gastritis, yellow fever and tuberculosis are some of the diseases where such campaigning methods have become successful. Pharmacist can participate and use his knowledge in such campaigning. Advertisement regarding discovery of vaccine for viral diseases have brought a new hope for future. Considerable development in chemotherapy and chemoprophylaxis has lead to a significant control on diseases like tuberculosis and leprosy. Community pharmacist has a much role in advertisement of such development so that patient will get a long lasting treatment and get rid of it. Community pharmacy can take over a significant role in surveillance in the epidemiological surveillance consists of continuous scrutiny of distribution and spread of infection, prediction of the development of potentially dangerous situation and collection of data for effective control of it.

Health education in the area of food hygiene mainly deals with food obtained from animal source such as milk, meat, poultry and fish. It also deals with nutritional value assessment, hygiene, storage and handling of food material. This includes a special aspect in microbiological point of view. The work includes development of laboratory methods for food examination. Developments of simple, rapid and cost effective techniques are for routine analysis and quality control examination. Pharmacist as analytical expert has a significant role to play.

Polypharmacy

Polypharmacy is a use of multiple medications due to multiple medical conditions. This is more evident in geriatric patient where multiple medical conditions arise as a matter of age for example, hypertension, arthritis, diabetes in this conditions a multiple drug treatment from more than one physician leads to polypharmacy. Polypharmacy more precisely can be defining as administration of more medicine than a clinical indication and requirement representing unnecessary drug utilization. Use of multiple drug increases risk of drug-drug interaction, non-adherence to drug therapy, adverse effects and higher cost of treatment. Although polypharmacy is the issue related to geriatric patients it is also issue amongst general population.

Polypharmacy may be result of too many prescriptions of drugs for the same clinical condition of the same patient, too many number of different dosage form making it confused and multiple administration of same drug, a part of treatment is no evidence based, use of two or more drugs from same medical class, multiple disease conditions in same patient (especially in geriatric patients), multiple doctors prescribing for same patient, change in physician without stopping the treatment of previous physician, multiple filling of prescription from different pharmacy, lack of patient education etc. Polypharmacy may not be problematic if multiple drug administration does not lead to a significant side effect. Such multiple drug treatment is necessary in many conditions. Polypharmacy however become problematic when negative outcome occurs resulting in to unnecessary and inappropriate medication prescription, increased risk for drug interaction and adverse drug reactions, non-adherence and increase expenditures of the treatment.

Prescribing inappropriate medicines also often results into polypharmacy. For example, a patient receiving amitriptyline for the treatment of insomnia results into a side effect as constipation, urinary incontinence, dizziness, dry mouth, dry eyes etc., to treat this side effect secondary medicine may be prescribed as laxatives, diuretics and eye drop. The prescription for the treatment of insomnia landed into total 4 drugs to patient.

Treatment for polypharmacy includes maintenance of accurate record and medical history, linking each prescribed medicine for disease, identifying medications that are for the treatment of side effects, intervention for patience adherence, reconciliation of drug treatment on discharge from hospital and appropriate preventive measures.

The role of the pharmacist in the prevention and treatment of polypharmacy is depending on the health care system. In geriatric patient long term treatment can be monitored by pharmacist. Using counseling technique the patient's adherence can be improved. In hospital pharmacy reviewing and prescription for complete and accurate medication will reduce the risk of polypharmacy. Community pharmacist can prevent the incidences of polypharmacy by preventing dispensing of unnecessary, inappropriate and side effect prone drugs.

References

2012 FIP Global Pharmacy; Workforce Report; www.fip.org

A.J. Winfield, R.M.E. Richards (2004). Pharmaceutical Practice, 3rd edition, Churchill Livingstone.

Andrew W Joyce, V Bruce Sunderland, Suzanne Burrows, Alexandra McManus, Peter Howat, Bruce Maycock (2007). Community Pharmacy's Role in Promoting Healthy Behaviours. *Journal of Pharmacy Practice and Research* **37(1):** 42-44.

Benoit Rouleau, Louise Lavoie, Jacinthe Leblanc, Simon Moretti, Chantal Collin (2011). Reporting of Adverse Drug Reactions by Community Pharmacists: A Qualitative Study in Quebec. *Drug Information Journal* **45:** 627-639.

Chijioke O. Agomo (2012). The role of community pharmacists in public health: a scoping review of the literature. *Journal of Pharmaceutical health Service Research* **3:** 25-33.

Cooper and Gunn (1987). Dispensing for Pharmaceutical Students, 12th edition, CBS publishers and distributors.

D.W. Bates, D.L. Boyle, N. Laird *et al.,* (1995). Incidence of Adverse Drug Events and Potential Adverse Drug Events. *J.A.M.A.* **274:** 29-34.

Emily R. Hajjar, Angela C. Cafiero and Joseph T. Hanlon. Polypharmacy in Elderly Patients. *The American Journal of Geriatric Pharmacotherapy* **5(4):** 345-351.

FIP Reference Guide on Good Pharmacy Practice in Community and Hospital settings, International Pharmaceutical Federation, PO Box 84200, 2508 AE The Hague, The Netherlands, 1st edition (2009), 1-62.

Guidance for Hospitals, Nursing Homes, and Other Health Care Facilities; U.S. Department of Health and Human Services, Food and Drug Administration, Center for Drug Evaluation and Research (CDER), (March 2001); Compliance.

Habeeb Ibrahim AR, Deepak Jose and Jegan RS (2012). Pharmacists in the Wider Public Health Workforce - A Review. *Archives of Pharmacy Practice* **3(2):** 166-169.

http://bostonabcd.org/community-health-education.aspx

http://brown.edu

http://epi.publichealth.nc.gov

http://www.cisco-eagle.com

http://www.ehow.com/list_6596347_duties-community-pharmacist.html

http://www.en.wikipedia.org

http://www.fda.gov/cder/guidance/index.htm

http://www.gatesfoundation.org/familyplanning/Pages/overview.aspx

http://www.health.ny.gov

http://www.healthed.ca

http://www.healtheducation.uci.edu/tobacco/tobacco.aspx

http://www.medicinenet.com

http://www.ncbi.nlm.nih.gov

http://www.pharmacy.purdue.edu/students/prospective/Responsibilities.php

http://www.psnc.org.uk/pages/about_community_pharmacy.html

Institute for safe medication practice; www.ismp.org

Kirsten K. Viktil, Hege S. Blix, Tron A. Moger, Aasmund Reikvam (2006). Polypharmacy as commonly defined is an indicator of limited value in the assessment of drug-related problems; *British Journal of Clinical Pharmacology* **63(2):** 187-195.

L.L. Leape, D.W. Bates, D.J. Cullen *et al.*, (1995). Systems Analysis of Adverse Drug Events. *J.A.M.A.* **274:** 35-43.

N.K. Jain, S.N. Sharma (1997). A text book of Professional Pharmacy, 4th edition, Vallabh Prakashan, New Delhi.

Priyanka V Patil, Ashwin Mali, Ashwin Kuchekar, Atmaram Pawar (2011). The future of prescription: e-prescription. *International Journal of Community Pharmacy* **(4)2:** 14-18.

Remington (2005). The Science and Practice of Pharmacy, 21st edition, Lippincott Williams & Wilkins.

Satya P. Krishnan (1996). Health Education at Family Planning Clinics: Strategies for Improving Information about Contraception and Sexually Transmitted Diseases for Low-Income Women. *Health Communication* **8(4):** 353-366.

CHAPTER 3

Dispensing Pharmacy

Definition

Dispensing is the compounding and supply of medicine by the pharmacist/druggist or under the supervision of pharmacist as per the legal prescription of the medical practitioner for individual patient or hospital to ensure safe and effective use of medicine by the patient. It also involves interpretation, evaluation and implement-tation of prescription after receiving, selection, manipulation and compounding of medicine, selection of suitable container, labeling and supply of product. All the above acts must be done as per the regulatory guidelines and requirement under a strict controlled environment. Pharmacist involved in dispensing should be a registered pharmacist as per the regulatory requirement. His/her name should be in the register of Pharmacy Council of India constituted as per Pharmacy Act 1948 in the state where his pharmacy shop is present. The dispensing of medicines involves both technical and cognitive components. Receiving and reading prescription, selecting drug to dispense, checking the expiry date, labeling, and final physical checking are the technical tasks. Assessment of therapeutic appropriateness, recommendation to prescriber and advising to the patients are the cognitive components. Administrations of substance by injection or inhalation, applying topically are not included in the dispensing process.

For the effective dispensing the pharmacist must have a thorough knowledge of medicine in relation to its stability, efficacy, safety profile, dose, route of administration, therapeutic index, contra-indications, incompatibility issues, packing and labeling, storage condition, record keeping and other regulatory requirements etc. To understand above things pharmacist must study the pharmaceutics, pharmachemistry, pharmacology, forensic pharmacy, pharmacognosy-identification of plants and other naturally occurring substances (including Ayurveda, Unani, Siddha, Homeopathy etc.) which are used to treat the diseases. The knowledge of pharmaceutics will help pharmacist for compounding and dispensing of the dosage form, chemistry will give idea about chemical nature, incompatibility issue, storage and handling of the substances, knowledge of pharmacology is necessary to know therapeutic efficacy, therapeutic index, side effect and forensic pharmacy will give an idea about legal requirement like container, labeling, storage, record keeping and ethical practice etc. Along with these main stream subject pharmacist must have knowledge of other subjects like clinical pharmacy, microbiology, pharmacognosy, pathology etc., local and communication languages and skills.

Guidelines for Dispensing

Implementation of good dispensing procedure is a vital for ensuring the errors that are detected and corrected at all the stages during process. The use of written document as a standard operating procedure and implementation of good dispensing practice will improve consistency and quality of work.

Receiving, Reading and Checking Prescription

A prescription received by patient or from online computer system. Pharmacist is responsible for confirmation of all the legal and other aspects of the prescription. Pharmacist should confirm the name and other details of the patient first. This stage is required in pharmacy where large crowd may be present, where everybody needs urgent attention for their prescription. Pharmacist has to speed up the process with accuracy. This will avoid mix up of prescription, dispensing the prescription to other patient etc. cross-checking of name and identity of patient must be done during issuing the medicine most care should be taken also. Upon confirmation the prescription should be read carefully and understood. The pharmacist should read the prescription and correctly interpret the abbreviations and Latin terms used in the prescription. He should not show any facial expressions so as to create any doubt in mind of patient. He should check the dose prescribed for the particular person. By asking few questions to patient he may confirm the nature of disorder symptoms if necessary. By virtue of his knowledge he should check any kind of drug-drug interaction in the prescribed medicine and any kind of drug-food interaction and if such drug-food interaction found, patient should be clearly instructed during giving instructing of dosing. A special precaution must be taken during dispensing the pediatric prescription. The pharmacist must refer in to the special posology terms used in it.

Compounding

On confirmation, reading, checking and understanding the prescription, pharmacist must perform the calculation if necessary before starting the compounding process. The calculation may be necessary for amount of drug/excipients to be taken, total quantity to be dispensed etc. During dispensing it is assumed that pharmacist has already checked the prescription for its legal aspect and correctness. Pharmacist should use his experience and conscious to handle such situations and in such case order should be sent back in written form to ensure accuracy for dispensing. All calculations must be double checked for correctness or should be counterchecked by another person. An arithmetic error may become fatal to the health of patient. The calculations must be recorded in prescription compounding register.

Preparation of dosage form for issue to the patient is central part of dispensing process. It should have a stepwise procedure depending on dosage form. The procedure should include stepwise ingredients taking and mixing by adopting appropriate procedure. It helps pharmacist for self checking and counter checking to ensure accuracy during process of formulating dosage form. This part of dispensing should after clear understanding of the prescription and checking calculation of the quantity of ingredients to be taken. It is good practice to have a stepwise checklist and preserving it with other record.

A good dispenser uses the first-in/first-out strategy during dispensing process. He selects the item by reading the label and cross matching the product name and strength, should check the stock and make sure that it should not expire. He should select the oldest stock first for dispensing. In any case he should not dispense expired stock. Depending on stock rotation method pharmacist read the label of all containers deliberately during dispensing process. Pharmacist should use proper weighing techniques for measuring the ingredients. During dispensing selecting the container of the ingredient according to color or location, without active and conscious reading the label is bad practice and may leads to fatal consequences. Opening many containers of same ingredient is another bad practice during dispensing. Ingredient may be double selected, another ingredient may be selected or some ingredient may overlook during dispensing process. Moreover the open containers are prone for deterioration due to unnecessary exposure to air.

During measuring the liquid ingredients a clean vessel must be used. Liquid should be poured from stock bottle, keeping the label upward to avoid spillage of liquid on the label which could dame it. Tablets and capsules can be counted without assistance of special device. A precaution must be taken that hand operation should not be used for counting process. It's a bad practice both in terms of hygienic and product quality reasons. Counting is done with help of piece of paper, knife, and spatula. Specially designed tablet counting device, lid of stock container or any clean and dust free surface may be used to count the tablets and capsules.

Immediately after the measurement or counting the stock container lid should be replaced and label of container should be checked once again for the medicine name. The stock container should be replaced in its original position. One of the good practice busy pharmacists can undertake is that prepackaging of widely/frequently used medicine.

Packing and Labeling

A medicament after compounding should be packed in a suitable container so that it can be easy for handling and storage by the patient. Container should be clean, dry, and suitable to undertake pouring/removal and measurement/counting of dosage form. Container itself should not affect the quality of medicine in any way. The dosage form is packed in containers like glass/plastic bottle, paper/plastic envelop, cardboard box etc. The container should be suitable so as to protect the drug from environmental condition till its shelf life. During humid environment the cardboard box may not be appropriate to protect dosage form and in those days a plastic lined boxes may be useful.

The purpose of container is to protect the medicine till its shelf life from variable environmental and handling condition during administration. The container also provides a surface area for writing the details of medicine and other information of patients use like instructions, route, dose and frequency of administration. The container and closure would meet certain standards, which include nature and color of container and closure, good labeling practice etc. The tablets and capsules are packed in clean, dry, glass or plastic bottle with tight fitted cap or seals and should protect the medicine form dirt and moisture. Blister packages, tight sealing glass or plastic containers with screw or snip cap, zip locked plastic bags or tin with tight-fitting closure are ideal containers for tablet and capsules. For the liquid dosage forms (oral or topical) the container must be clean, dry, light resistant, glass or plastic, with leak proof tight fitting closure or cap. An amber color or opaque, glass or plastic bottle with screw or snip tight fitting cap are suitable. Many times the cap of container is provided as a measuring device. Dosage forms are measure in cap. For semisolid preparations like cream or ointments clean glass or porcelain wide mouth containers or jars are used. It should be provided with tight fitted lid of plastic or metal. A metal or plastic collapsible tube with cap is also used for semisolid preparation.

Under any circumstance two similar or different dosage forms should not be packed in single container. Two liquids should not be mixed together in any case. Even if tablets or capsules have different size, shape, colors as identification criteria they should be packed in different containers as the direction of their administration may be different. Mixing two dosage forms might interact with each other physically or chemically. A specially designed device for helping patients (elder or having forgetful mind) and containing complex medication regimens are available now a days. These containers typically hold the medicine for using seven days/fifteen days etc. The reminder of container gives an idea about dosage administered, missing dose if any.

Physical Checking of Finished Product

At this stage dispensed preparation should be checked once again for reading, interpretation, calculations, dispensing, check for appropriate dosage prescribed and drug interaction, identity of medicine dispensed, suitability of container, labels and countersign of pharmacist. This step can be done by pharmacist or another staff member. It is advisable that physical checking of finished product should be done by another staff member.

Record Keeping

Record keeping of dispensed product is essential for effective management of dispensary, for verification of stock used in dispensing, for back tracking of dispensed product if any complications arise and as a legal requirement. Various methods are used for record keeping. Prescriptions dispensed will be retained by pharmacist and appropriate annotation with strength and quantity of each medicine dispensed will be recorded with each prescription. These prescriptions are then filled or details be entered in record book. The information must contain patient's details like name, age, gender, address, etc., the details of medicine contains medicine name, strength and quantity etc. Entry of dispensers name is must in order to keep accountability of dispensing. In many modern pharmacies the use of computer software has ease the record keeping of dispensed prescriptions. The information entered in computer software can be recalled for generation of summary, stock maintenance, account etc.

After appropriate record keeping the medicine are issued to the patients with instructions regarding when to take medicine, how to take medicine and how to store medicine. Warning regarding side effect must be given with caution because it may affect patient's adherence, and may create frightening and patient stops taking medicine. Every effort is made to confirm that patient understood the instructions clearly.

As per Australian Incident Monitoring System around 10% of the medication incidences occur as a result of dispensing errors and as per the suggestions of US National Academy of Science 78% errors can be avoided by automated dispensing system. The most common errors in dispensing are selection of incorrect strength and selection of incorrect product. The major contributing factors are they look-alike and they sound-alike. High dispensing of prescription volume and interruptions are also contributing factors in it. This all can be minimized using automation. In channel storage system stock is manually loaded into predetermined location. In random storage, robotics can be used where the packs are stored according to diminutions for effective utilization of space. The robotics selects the location of correct dispensing and minimizes the errors occurring during dispensing. The robotic dispensing reduces dispensing errors, staff can be released from dispensing to patients care, reduce stock holding, improves stock rotation, fasten the dispensing process, on call working and have an improved space utilization.

Classification and Dispensing of Dosage Forms

A dosage form is preparation which may contain active drug molecule so as to deliver that molecule at the site of action within the body. The therapeutic efficacy of drug depends on the amount of drug reaches at the site of action in a specified amount. The dose of drug depends on the route by which dosage form is administered; nature of barriers to reach the drug at site and nature of drug itself. The bioavailability of dosage form largely depends on route of administration, nature of dosage form, release of drug from dosage form and crossing of biological membrane by drug. Along with therapeutic effect, drugs also produce side effects which are undesirable. The side effects of drugs can be minimized by reducing the dose of drug without sacrificing the therapeutic effect. This can be achieved by formulating the drug in appropriate dosage form intended for medicinal use. The suitability of drug molecule for the particular dosage form and patients needs are important issues taken in account during selection of dosage form to be formulated. Depending upon the route of administration type of dosage forms can be classified as follows. The dosage forms are typically used for particular route of administration but it's not true always. Many type of dosage forms are may be used by more than one route of administration. For example, solutions and powders are predominantly used for oral route but topical solutions and powders are also available.

Topical

- Collodions
- Creams
- Dusting powders
- Emulsions
- Gels
- Liniments
- Lotions
- Ointments
- Poultices
- Sprays
- Paints
- Pastes

Oral

- Aromatic waters
- Cachets
- Capsules
- Elixirs
- Extracts
- Gargles
- Linctuses
- Lozenges
- Mixtures
- Mouthwashes
- Oral emulsions
- Oral liquids
- Powder for mixtures
- Solution tablets
- Solutions
- Spirits
- Syrups

- Glycerites
- Granules
- Infusions
- Oral powders
- Pastilles
- Pills
- Tablets
- Tinctures

Parenteral

- Injectables
- Implants
- Irrigations
- Insufflations
- Parenteral preparations

Inhalations

- Aerosols
- Inhalations
- Vitrellae

Rectal

- Enemas
- Suppositories

Other

- Ear drops
- Eye drops
- Eye lotions
- Eye ointments
- Medical gases
- Nasal drops
- Nasal sprays
- Pessaries
- Surgical dressings

- **Aerosols:** Aerosols are pressurized dosage form containing active medicament with propellant, to aid the delivery in fine mist form. The medicament may in the form of fine powder of liquid particles. The aerosols are typically used for respiratory or topical application. For example, aerosol of salbutamol, corticosteroids for asthmatic patient or a pain killer aerosol containing methyl salicylate for topical application. The aerosol has two types of designs depending on mechanism of operation. A pressurized container contains propellant which delivers contents upon pressing the actuator, while a nebulizer device delivers contents with the help of mechanical pumping action of actuator. A pressurized delivery system with metered actuator regulates delivery of recommended quantity of medicament at each dose.
- **Aromatic waters:** Aromatic waters are clear, aqueous, saturated solutions of volatile liquid, volatile medicaments or aromatic substances. Their flavor is similar to that of drug or volatile substance. They are mainly used for flavoring agents for

medicament, as a vehicle and diluents. They also exert mild carminative action.

- **Cachets:** These are used to dispense nauseous or disagreeable powders in a tasteless form. A medium density powder up to 2 gm can be dispensed in a modulated rice paper wafer as a single dose. They are soften, using water, before administration and then taken as draught of water. Now a day's cachets are not dispensed.
- **Capsules:** capsule is solid dosage form in which a medicament is enclosed in a shell of gelatin (hard or soft) intended for oral administration. Like cachets a drug with nauseous or disagreeable test or powder which cannot be formulated in other dosage form like tablet are encapsulated. Capsules are of two type, hard gelatin and soft gelatin. Hard gelatin capsules are used for dispensing solid powder or granules. It consists of two parts, cylindrical body and cap. It is available in variable sizes from 000 (largest) to 5 (smallest). Soft gelatin capsule are one piece capsule suitable for solid, semisolid, suspension or liquids. They are formed filled and sealed in sequential single stage manufacturing process. Soft gelatin capsule contains glycerin as plasticizer which gives flexibility to the shell. Capsule dosage form is swallowed as a whole with water. Soft surface facilitates its administration. Gelatin shell dissolves in gastric content of stomach and release medicament immediately.
- **Collodions:** Collodions are liquid preparation for external use for application to skin. They are applied with special applicant like brush. It contains volatile vehicle such as ether or ethanol. Upon application to skin, vehicle evaporates and leaves a thin protective and flexible film on skin for prolongs contact between skin and medicament.
- **Creams:** Creams are semisolid emulsions for external use. Depending on continuous phase they are either aqueous or oily. Aqueous cream emulsions are of oil-in-water type and oily cream emulsions are of water-in-oil type. Oil-in-water creams are non-greasy in nature. Creams exert emollient or moisturizing effect on skin and also used for percutaneous delivery of drugs.
- **Dusting powders:** Dusting powers are used for external use. It's a very fine free flowing powder. It may contain medicaments. Powder has greater specific surface area. Drugs are dispensed in

powder dosage form. Dusting powders are not used for open wound unless they are sterilized. Kaolin is used as diluents. Antiseptic, antibacterial substances are incorporated in it.

- **Ear drops:** Ear drops are solutions, suspensions, emulsions or any form of liquid preparation intended for instillation into the ear using dropper. The vehicles used for ear drops contain water, glycerol, polypropylene glycol or alcohol. Almond oil, Olive oil are used for impacted earwax.
- **Elixirs:** Elixirs are oral preparation. They are pleasantly flavored clear liquid preparation containing potent or nauseous medicament. Elixirs are more stable than mixtures. They contain attractive coloring agent, ethanol and syrup, glycerol, propylene glycol together as a vehicle and antimicrobial as a preservative. Sugar free vehicle such as sorbitol is also used. The drugs which are unstable in liquid dosage form and to be given by oral to pediatric patients are formulated as elixirs. In a bottle dry granules or powder is supplied which is formulated before administration.
- **Emulsions:** Emulsions are oral or topical dosage form like creams. They are thermodynamically unstable system consisting of mixture of two immiscible liquids. One of which is oil and another is water or aqueous phase. One phase is dispersed in another. The phase dispersed as a globule is called as dispersed phase and phase in which dispersion is made is known as continuous phase. The presence of emulsifying agent stabilizes this system. Depending on dispersed phase and continuous phase emulsion can be subcategorized as:
    1. Oil in water (o/w) emulsion.
    2. Water in oil (w/o) emulsion.
    3. Multiple (o/w/o or w/o/w) emulsion and
    4. Microemulsion.

  In o/w emulsion oil phase is dispersed as globules in aqueous continuous phase. When oil phase is continuous phase and aqueous phase is in the form of globules then emulsion is termed as w/o emulsion. In multiple emulsions continuous phase emulsion is dispersed in another phase as droplets. Microemulsions are homogeneous transparent system of low viscosity. It contains high percentage of both oil and aqueous phase.

- **Enemas:** Enemas are intended for rectal administration. They are oily or aqueous solutions, suspension or emulsions containing medicaments for local treatment like ulcerative colitis or x-ray contrast media. Some drugs like diazepam can also be administered rectally in the form of enemas for systemic absorption and effect for the treatment of epilepsy where patient cannot take drug voluntarily.
- **Extracts:** Extracts are mostly aqueous concentrated preparations containing active ingredients from plant or animal origin. The active principles are extracted using suitable solvents and solvents are evaporated till a concentrated solution or soft mass is formed. Extracts are used as oral preparation or topical applicants or it can be a part of other preparation.
- **Eye drops:** Eye drops are sterile preparation used for instillation in to the conjunctival sac of eye. Eye drops may be solutions or suspensions of one or more than one medicament. They are generally packed in single dose or multiple dose containers and supplied with separate dropper fitted on container.
- **Eye lotions:** Eye lotions are used as a first aid for cleaning eyes. They are sterile aqueous solutions and used as it is. It does not contain any bactericidal agent. The eye lotions must be used within 24 hr after opening the container.
- **Eye ointments:** Eye ointments are sterile semi-solid preparation for instillation in to conjunctiva or eyelid. They contain one or more medicament dispersed in nonirritant ointment base. Eye ointments are packed in single gelatin applicaps or multi-dose small volume metal or plastic collapsible tubes.
- **Gargles:** Gargles are aqueous solutions used for local action on throat. They are used in prevention and treatment of throat infections. They are prepared and dispensed as concentrated solutions of medicament and patients are instructed to dilute it with water before use. Gargles should not be swallowed and should be spit out after a minute of treatment on throat.
- **Gels:** Gels are semisolid preparation for topical applications. They are translucent or transparent, non-greasy, aqueous, colloidal suspension of insoluble or soluble medicament. Gels contain gelling agents like gelatin, starch, tragacanth, sodium

alginate, cellulose etc. They may be sterile preparation if intended for application to open wounds. The term gel is also applicable to colloidal solution of aluminum and magnesium hydroxide which is used as an antacid.

- **Glycerites:** Glycerites are viscous solutions of medicament in glycerol with or without water, prepared with or without heating intended for oral administration. They are generally used as antiseptics or anti-inflammatory.
- **Granules:** Granules are oral dosage forms. They are small irregular particles of around 2 mm diameter and supplied in a single dose sachet or bulk container where the dose is measured using spoon. Granules contain sugar, flavoring agents and inert adjuncts along with medicaments. Granules are placed on tongue and swallowed with water or dissolved in water before taking. Effervescent granules are mixture of citric acid, tartaric acid and sodium bicarbonate along with medicament and sweetening agent. They evolve carbon dioxide when added to water.
- **Implants:** Implants are sterile solid dosage form. Sterile disks or cylinders are implanted surgically inside the body tissues or inserted under the skin for sustain release of medicaments for prolong period of time. They are generally used for hormonal replacement therapy and contraceptives.
- **Infusions:** Infusions are made by fresh extractions of drugs obtained from plant source in cold or boiling water. The method is no longer used for medicinal purpose because infusions support the microbial growth. Hence every time fresh infusions are made. Infusions are now a day's replaced with extracts. Infusions are used for oral as well as topical application depending on medicinal plant extract.
- **Inhalations:** Inhalations are liquid preparation containing volatile substances intended for nasal/mouth use. They are used for the treatment of upper respiratory tract infection/diseases. The medicaments used in inhalations are volatile at room temperature and are inhaled using handkerchief or fabric cloth mask. The liquids can also be used with water vaporizers for steam inhalation. The inhalation liquid may be enclosed in soft gelatin capsule, it may be a readymade liquid to be added to hot water (not boiling) or it may be a simple solution dissolved in alcoholic solvent. Over use of inhalations should be avoided as

they may cause chronic conditions. Now a day's they are in the form of capsule which will be broken at the time of inhalation and it will be inhaled by mouth with vapourizer.

- **Injectables:** Injectables are synonymously known as parenteral preparations. They deliver the medicine to patients other than alimentary canal. These are sterile dosage forms containing one or more medicaments or electrolyte for replacements. These dosage forms are administered using aseptic techniques and special appliances like syringe, needles, and infusion set etc. Parenteral route is used when drug cannot be given by oral route by any reason. Patients intolerance, poor gastric solubility of drug, degradation of medicament in gastric pH, instability of drug in oral dosage forms, poor absorption of drug, localization of effect, unconscious patients, rapid administration of fluid, ensure targeted delivery of drug are some of the reasons for giving drug parenterally. Injection is directly enters in blood vessel or a particular tissue, tissue space or body compartment using suitable device by expert person to do so. With advancement of technology of injectables are manufactured, and such injections can be given without hospital or clinical environment. Patients can use it at home, at workplace, allowing them administered themselves with a short training session. Parenteral formulations are directly administered into blood for fast and controlled effect and in to tissue outside the blood vessel for local or systemic effect.

- **Insufflations:** Insufflation is dosage form designed to present drug in dry powder form packed in capsule and delivered by a special device known as insufflators. The powder is blown in to ear, nose, throat or other body cavity where the application of powder is difficult. The capsule containing powder is broken in to the insufflators and released drug is inhaled by patient or blown in the cavity of patient.

- **Irrigation solutions:** Irrigation solutions are sterile, pyrogen free solutions used for bath, flush, irrigation of body cavities, operation cavity, wound, nose, ear, throat or urogenital system. They are always used topically and never given parenterally. Irrigation solutions contain plain saline (0.9% NaCl) or may contain some antibacterial or antifungal agent. The main purpose of irrigation solution is to clean the infections of body cavities. They are administered using soft catheter and removed back.

- **Linctuses:** Linctuses are viscous liquid preparations intended for oral use in the treatment of cough. They are simple solution containing high proportion of syrup, sucrose, and glycerol which have demulcent action and effect on mucous membrane of throat. Linctuses are taken undiluted in a prescribed dose. It should be sipped slowly and swallowed neatly so as to produce prolonged contact between linctuses and throat.
- **Liniments:** Liniments are used for external application to skin for alleviate discomfort of muscle strains and injury. They are liquid, semi-liquid or semi-solid preparations. They are alcoholic, oily solutions or emulsions containing medicament. Liniments are massaged on skin and provide counter irritant, stimulant, rubefacient action depending on ingredients in it. They may be applied with warm dressings. Liniments are never applied to broken skin.
- **Lotions:** Lotions are externally used liquid preparations. They may be solutions, suspensions or emulsions. They are dabbed on skin or applied with suitable dressing. They are used as antiseptic, soothing, parasiticidal. Lotions have many similar characteristics like cream. Lotions are fluid and can be poured while creams cannot.
- **Lozenges:** Lozenges are also known as troches. They are semisolid large tablets designed so that they remain in mouth for around 15 min and sucked. The main purpose of lozenges is to treat mouth and throat infection. It is sugar and gum base. Sugar provides sweet taste during sucking and gum gives strength, cohesiveness and facilitates slow release of medicament for local action in mouth and on throat for cough remedies.
- **Medical gases:** Medical gases are products that are directly administered as gases. They have direct therapeutic action and used as diluents for other medicated gas. They can also be used for aerosol administration as an adjunct. They may be single component or mixture of two or more gases. These gases are stored in compressed cylinders. Medical gases are administered *via* pulmonary route using regulator and metered flow controlled device as delivery system for regulation of rate and volume of gas under ambient temperature and pressure conditions.

- **Mixtures:** Mixtures are aqueous oral preparations containing one or more medicaments in solution or suspension form. They are formulated for short life span and do not have long shelf-life. It should be freshly and recently prepared and used quickly within month.
- **Mouthwashes:** Mouthwash is similar to gargles they are used to maintain mouth hygiene and for treatment of mouth infections. The active ingredients are usually antiseptics and antibacterial.
- **Nasal drops:** Nasal drops are isotonic solutions for instillation into nose using dropper. Drug has local action on nasal mucosa like decongestant, vasoconstriction, antihistaminic effect etc. Other preparation may contain hormones like oxytocin, vasopressin which are delivered through nasal mucosa. The bottle containing nasal drop is supplied with dropper device to allow patient for self-administration dose of drug.
- **Nasal sprays:** Nasal sprays are similar to that of nasal drop. They are formulated as sprays.
- **Ointments:** Ointments are semisolid, greasy preparations containing less than 20% water, volatile components and are intended for topical use like skin, mucosa, ophthalmic or rectum. They contain more than 50% hydrocarbon, waxes, polyols as a vehicle. The base is anhydrous and immiscible with skin secretions. They are used as emollients to make skin more pliable, protective barriers to prevent contact of harmful substances with skin, as a vehicle for incorporation of medicaments. Ointment used on open wounds should be sterile. Ointment contain four types of bases hydrocarbon base, absorption base, water removable base, water soluble base.
- **Oral emulsions:** Oral emulsions are o/w type of emulsion (as described previously) containing one or more medicament and intended for oral administration. The medicament may be a part of dispersed phase or continuous phase.
- **Oral liquids:** Oral liquids are liquid preparation for oral use containing one or more ingredients dissolved or suspended in vehicle. Elixirs, linctuses, mixtures, drops, oral emulsions, oral solutions, oral suspensions are all oral liquids.
- **Oral powders:** There are two types of oral powders used for oral administration. Bulk powder contains non-potent

medicaments like antacids, mucoprotectants, bulk enhancers etc. Powder is measured by spoon and dispersed in water and taken. Divided powders contains potent active medicament and are packed in individual sachets. Each dose is wrapped in separate piece of paper or sealed in sachet.

- **Paints:** Paints are liquids or solutions used for application to skin or mucosal membrane. Paints contain volatile liquids which on application to skin evaporate and leave a thin protective film on skin surface with active ingredient for prolonged action. Paints applied to mucus membrane of oral cavity or throat, contains viscous vehicles like glycerol. This forms a sticky and adhesive film of paint on mucous membrane for prolonged period of time and enables the preparation to remain in contact with affected area. The paints may contain medicaments for antiseptic, analgesic, astringent effect.
- **Parenteral preparations:** The term parenteral preparations and injectables are used synonymously.
- **Pastes:** Pastes are semisolid preparation for external application. They are similar to that of creams and ointments. They containing high proportion of finely grounded powder medicament (more than 25% w/w). The powders are formulated with anhydrous or water soluble base. Pastes are stiff in consistency and make them useful as a protective covering.
- **Pastilles:** Pastilles are solid dosage forms. They softer than lozenges. They contains glycerol-gelatin base. Pastilles dissolve slowly in mouth and contain medicaments like antiseptics, astringents, anesthetics etc., intended for relief of conditions affecting mouth and throat.
- **Pessaries:** Pessaries are medicated solid dosage forms intended for insertion into vagina. After insertion they melt or dissolved and release medicaments for local action or systemic absorption. Pessaries are of different types depending on manufacturing process. They are moulded in cone shape similar way to suppositories. Pessaries may be compressed as vaginal tablets in various sizes and shapes similar to oral tablets. Vaginal capsules are similar to soft gelatin oral capsules of different size and shapes.

- **Pills:** Pills are moulded, solid oral dosage forms. They consist of spherical masses containing one or more medicaments in it. Pills are rarely use now a days. The term pill is synonymously used for oral contraceptive tablets due to their shape.
- **Poultices:** Poultices are paste like preparation and has a heat bearing capacity intended for external application for treatment of conditions like inflammation. They are heated and applied on the affected surface area by spreading thickly with dressing. For example, kaolin poultice.
- **Powders for mixtures:** Powders for mixtures are powders mixed in proportions for preparation of suspensions. The proportionally mixed powder is stored in dry form and constituted before dispensing by adding sufficient water or vehicle in it. The final product dispensed by pharmacist is suspension intended for oral or topical application.
- **Solutions:** Solutions are liquid preparations intended for various purposes. They may be medicated or non-medicated. Medicated sterile solutions are used as injections, peritoneal dialysis, anticoagulants, irrigation fluids etc. Non-sterile medicated or non-medicated solutions are used as oral preparations or for topical applications.
- **Solution tablets:** Solution tablets are compressed dosage forms that are dissolved in water to produce solution which is used as above. These tablets are formulated for quick dissolution.
- **Spirits:** Spirits are alcoholic or hydro-aqueous solutions of volatile oils used as flavoring agents.
- **Sprays:** Sprays are alcoholic, aqueous or glycerol containing solutions of medicament applied to the mucosal membrane of nose, throat with the help of atomizer of aerosol.
- **Suppositories:** Suppositories are conical shaped semisolid or solid dosage form. They are intended for rectal administration. They contain medicaments for local or systemic actions. After insertion in to rectum suppository melt and release medicament for local action on rectal mucosa or medicament is absorbed in systemic circulation for effect.
- **Syrups:** Syrups are liquid preparations used as a vehicle for oral formulations. They are concentrated aqueous solutions of sucrose or other sugar. Flavored syrups are used for masking

disagreeable taste. Now a day's sugars have been replaced by sorbitol because of its dental problem on prolonged use. Syrup is synonymously used for sweet flavoring vehicle.

- **Tablets:** Tablet is solid dosage form usually intended for oral administration containing one or more medicaments. It is most widely used and popular dosage form. Tablets are available in various size, shapes and colors. Tablets are made by compressing medicaments with various other pharmaceutical excipients. Some tablets are prepared by moulding. Depending on mode of administration and techniques they are made, tablet can be of different types as vaginal, rectal, dispersible, effervescent, chewable, film coated, sugar coated, enteric coated, modified release, sustained release, sublingual, buccal etc. In addition to active pharmaceutical ingredient tablet also contains various excipients like diluents, binders, disintegrants, lubricants etc. Tablets are coated by various techniques like sugar coating, film coating to prevent environmental damage of medicament or for masking unpleasant flavor and taste. Enteric coated tablet resist dissolution and disintegration in stomach.
- **Tinctures:** Tinctures are alcoholic preparations of active principles from plant drugs. Tinctures are weak in relation to extract.
- **Vitrellae:** Vitrellae contains volatile ingredients for inhalation purpose. The volatile ingredients are encapsulated in thin walled glass capsule protected with absorbent cotton and fabric bag. The capsule is crushed to release the vapors for inhalation. Volatile nitrites for angina pectoris are formulated as vitrellae.

Incompatibility

Incompatibility is an undesirable reaction that occurs between drug and other drug or additives added or even container of the product leading to alteration in therapeutic efficacy or safety profile of drug. The reactions that occur are of three types, physical, chemical and therapeutic. Incompatibility is confused with drug interaction. Drug interaction is alteration in effect of drug due to influence of another substance (may be chemical or nutrient) leading to dosage form that is no more of use for patients. Drug interaction occurs inside the body and cannot be seen, however incompatibility reactions occurs during formulating the dosage form or its stores during shelf life.

Incompatibility reactions are visible and can be avoided. Incompatibility issues if ignored may lead to fatal effect or under effect of medicaments, which may land the patients in dangerous situations. Incompatibility may occur during formulation, manufacturing, packing, storage or administration of dosage form.

Physical incompatibility is a physical interaction between two components of dosage form that may lead to visible recognizable changes like precipitation, color change or haziness etc. Chemical incompatibility is a chemical reaction that occurs in two components of formulation and change is not necessarily visible. There may or may not be a clear visible evidence of chemical reaction leading to deterioration of dosage form. Therapeutic incompatibility is not a physical or chemical reaction in between components of formulation but there is undesirable therapeutic reaction leading to potentiating of therapeutic effect, destruction of effectiveness or occurrence of toxic effect to the patient. The summary incompatibility leads to synergism, antagonism or toxic effect.

Physical Incompatibility

A Physical incompatibility is a result of physical reaction between two components of the formulation. Physical incompatibility is due to immiscibility, insolubility, liqufaction, precipitation, complexation etc. This leads to non-uniformity of dosage and inaccuracy during dosing by the patients. The physical reaction leads to phase separation or precipitation (generally after dilution with other solvent like alcohol) due to change in relation between ionization, non-ionization and solubility. The pH value and pKa values are major responsible factors behind the physical interaction. The change in pH value leads to change in pH dependent solubility. Mixing of incompatible substances leads to change in pH value and may results into salting out or precipitation of components. The precipitation occurs when a relative quantity of other component is added which changes the buffer capacity of earlier. pH dependent precipitation is rapid and can be identified very easily. Furthermore, adsorption can be a phenomenon where active medicament may be immobilized and localized in certain area of formulation specifically inner surface of containers.

Immiscibility is one of the physical incompatibilities that occur during storage of dosage form. Oils are immiscible with water but the problem is overcome by emulsification. Addition of emulsifying agent stabilizes the oil component in aqueous phase or vice versa. Addition of spirits, concentrated waters and alcoholic solutions of volatile oils as a flavoring agents or high concentration of salts or electrolytes leads to phase separation in emulsions and creams.

Liquid preparation like suspension contains high proportion of insoluble solids in the form of powders. These powders act as thickening agent and give elegant appearance to the products. The insoluble powders having poor wetting property are dispensed using suitable suspending agent and make them deflocculated. Upon sedimentation these deflocculated suspension disperse readily on shaking the bottles. The addition of alcoholic extract to these deflocculated preparations leads to precipitation or loss of deflocculating property of suspending agent and upon standing the hard cake is formed which is indiffusible.

When certain low melting point solids are powdered together there liquefaction or soft mass formation takes place. The substances which have such behaviors are camphor, menthol, thymol, phenol, chloral hydrate etc. Medicaments such as sodium salicylate, aspirin, phenazone also bears similar behaviors. These are also known as eutectic substances. When such components are present in solid dosage form like powders their liquefaction leads to formation of damp masses and powder losses their flow property significantly.

The formulations containing complexing components like carbowax, phenol, salicylic acid, tannic acid losses elegancy and acceptance of these products. The complexation is due to hydrogen bonding between hydroxyl group and oxygen of polyether chain leading to physical incompatibility.

Chemical Incompatibility

A chemical incompatibility means the active medicament is chemically modified or degraded by chemical oxidation, reduction, hydrolysis or decomposition. These chemical changes can be manifested by precipitation, turbidity or change in color of formulation. As a consequence of chemical change there is decrease in chemical composition of active drug and/or toxic by-product may be formed. The chemical reaction can occur between drug and solvent, two drugs, drug and adjuvant, drug and container etc. The consequences of chemical incompatibility leads to damage to the patient from toxic product formed include embolism from crystallization, tissue irritation due to drastic change in pH or failure of substance to produce therapeutic efficacy.

The chemical reactions that occur in between two substances include oxidation, reduction, hydrolysis, polymerization, isomerization, decarboxylation, combination and formation of insoluble complex. Oxidation is loss of electron or addition of oxygen in to the chemical structure of substance. Reduction is adding of hydrogen atom to the molecule. When oxidation reaction occurs with oxygen present in air, spontaneously, it is known as auto-oxidation where as when oxidation occurs in the presence of catalyst like metals or impurities then this is known as pre-oxidation. The factors that influence these oxidation processes include presence of oxygen in the atmosphere of dosage form, light that cause photochemical reactions, elevated temperature accelerates the oxidative reactions. Each drug has its ideal pH for stability and change in this pH also affects stability and accelerate the oxidation reaction. Oxidation reaction occurs faster in liquid state than in solid state. Presence of metal ions acts as catalyst for oxidation reaction. Oxidation reactions occur faster in aqueous state than in organic state. Presence of unsaturated bonds in the chemical structure (double and triple bonds in oils) undergoes oxidation leading to saturation. The measures that can be taken to prevent oxidative reaction includes addition of antioxidants like vitamin E, vitamin C, chemicals like EDTA, benzalkonium chloride etc. Protection for formulation from light using dark containers, storage of formulation in dark place and packing formulation in light absorbing material, selection of suitable dosage form (preferred dosage form is capsule), pH maintenance using buffer, selection of suitable solvent, storage of formulation in low temperature, protection of formulation from atmospheric oxidation by use of tight close container and by replacing oxygen with nitrogen prevents oxidation. The medicaments that undergo oxidation include phenylephrine, adrenaline, noradrenaline, tetracyclines, oils and vitamins.

Hydrolysis is a chemical reaction in which water molecule is used to break covalent bond in the drug molecule and insertion of water molecule across it. In ionic hydrolysis the compound is broken down in to ions by use of water molecule. Ionic hydrolysis is reversible reaction and it takes place spontaneously. The covalent bond between ions of compound is broken. Weak acidic and weak basic drugs are affected by ionic hydrolysis like conversion of codeine phosphate into codeine and phosphate. Molecular hydrolysis is another process in which molecule itself is broken down and hence it must be prevented. It is slow but irreversible reaction like hydrolysis of aspirin to salicylic acid and acetic acid. The drugs having chemical groups like esters (benzocaine, procaine), amides (chloramphenicol, sulphonamide) and nitriles undergo hydrolysis. Presence of water, change in pH and high temperature accelerate the hydrolysis process. For protection of drug from hydrolysis, it should be protected from moisture, organic solvent should be used instead of aqueous, pH should be maintained using buffers. Complex formation and use of surfactant and reduction in solubility leading to formation of suspension rather than solution are some of other remedies.

In polymerization the monomers are bonded together to form long chain polymers. Formation of paraformaldehyde from formaldehyde at elevated temperature and formation of allergens at elevated temperature from ampicillin are examples of polymerization. Factors that influence polymerization process include temperature, light, solvent and pH.

Isomers are the different arrangement of atoms of molecules having identical molecular formula. Many drugs have two isomers and one of them have therapeutic efficacy while other may be less potent or inactive. In such cases conversion of one isomer to other will leads to loss of therapeutic efficacy of drug. Isomerization of one type in another is chemical reaction leading to incompatibility. In optical isomerism optically active compound is converted to less active isomer for example, L-adrenalin is converted to D-adrenaline by change of pH. L-adrenaline is therapeutically active. D-adrenaline has same physical properties and molecular formula but different arrangement of atoms. The same type of isomerism occurs in D-tubocurarine which is more active than L-tubocurarine. Geometric isomerism is expressed as *Cis* and *Trans*. *Cis* mean similar groups on same direction in molecule and *Trans* means in opposite direction. Most of the time *Cis*-isomer is more active than *Trans*, example Vitamin A. Factors like temperature, pH, and solvent accelerate the conversion of one isomer to other.

The formulation containing bicarbonates may undergo decarboxylation reaction leading to formation and evolution of carbon dioxide gas. High temperature, pH and solvent influences for decarboxylation process. Formulations containing sodium bicarbonate are therefore not sterilized using high temperature or autoclaving. The drug like tetracyclines forms a complexation with divalent metal ions like calcium and forms complex which are insoluble. This complex formation due to chemical reaction between drug and metal ions leads to incompatibility and loss of therapeutic efficacy.

Therapeutic Incompatibility

Therapeutic incompatibility is change in therapeutic effect or response from that intended to one or more drugs when co-administered in the patient. Therapeutic incompatibility is within realm of physician and mainly related to the change in effects after administration of dosage form. Any change in therapeutic effect, occurrence of adverse drug reactions is considered to be a therapeutic incompatibility. This type of incompatibility can be predicted by the pharmacist using his knowledge and experience and should consult to the physician before dispensing the prescription. The therapeutic incompatibility includes errors in dosage, wrong dose or dosage form, prescription of contraindicated drugs in same prescription, synergistic and antagonistic drug prescription simultaneously etc. The therapeutic incompatibility may be intentional of unintentional.

Errors in doses are most serious type of therapeutic incompatibility, which occurs due to overdosing of medication. Pharmacist should take due care during dispensing of such prescription where the chances of dose errors can be there. Poor handwriting, busy physician, overlooked prescriptions are some of the factors that may lead to dose error. The quantity of drug dispensed may be more than the maximum dose recommended for particular drug. In the modern practice many drugs are available in different strengths and dosage forms. In such conditions the chances of dose errors can be there.

Many drugs have similarity in their names but their dosages are quite different. Different formulation may have similarity in name but different in the drug content. This may leads to a wrong dose or dosage form. For example, similarity in name can leads to selection of wrong drug like prednisone and prednisolone, digoxin and digitoxin. The drugs are available in different dosage forms and if dosage form is not clearly mentioned chances of dispensing wrong dosage form may be there. Pharmacist should seek clarification if doubtful about dispensing of prescriptions.

Prescription of contraindicated drugs, allergic drugs in certain disease condition or patients leads to therapeutic incompatibility. Prescription of corticosteroids is contraindicated to the patients having peptic ulcer problem. Atropine for the treatment of loose motion is contraindicated if patient is suffering from deficiency of lachrymal secretions. Administrating the synergistic or antagonistic drug may be deliberate of mistaken leading to therapeutic incompatibility. Co-administration of penicillin with probenecid prolongs the therapeutic efficacy of penicillin. This is a deliberate administration for beneficial effect hence example of intentional incompatibility. Simultaneous administration of potassium sparing diuretics and ACE inhibitors, adrenaline and phenoxybenzamine may be mistaken and gives sub-therapeutic effect of drug, is the example of unintentional incompatibility.

Weights and Measures

From as early as 4000 BC balance is used in the form of equal arm beam. The accuracy is based on the idea of stick and pans. During the 16th century knife-edge pivots were introduced and era of beam ends. Until the mid 19th century pharmacist were using the hand scale for compounding and dispensing of medicines. More accurate and convenient pillar mounted bench top weighing machine replaces hand operated techniques.

The first weights were stones. Original Mediterranean weights were seeds of liquorice. In ancient Greece lead was also used as weights. Romans evolved the English weights system using grain as a standard. Apothecaries' weight was used in Europe for measurement of pharmaceutical ingredients from early 1270. Elizabeth I decided that 7000 grains equal to 1 pound (Avoirdupois pound) used for selling of goods. However Henry VIII uses Troy weight of 5760 equal to 1 pound to test coins. Troy weights were generally used in prescribing and measuring despite of adaptation of avoirdupois system of measurement. The British pharmacopoeia 1914 adopted metric system for medicinal doses, while dispensing using Apothecaries system continue till 1971. London pharmacopoeia 1618 adopted Roman gallon as its basic liquid measurement system and gives the guidelines of conversion of liquid unit into Apothecary weight.

In the later era industrialization brought many changes in world and so in the measurement system also. A single unit of measurement was not sufficient and defining the larger and smaller unit becomes the need of time. The apothecary or Avoirdupois system has that limitations and make the calculations more complicated. The Arabic number system using base 10 was accepted worldwide as measurement system. Using the base 10 allows simple mathematics and conversion in between different units of measurement. The multiplication or division by 10 again and again makes the larger or smaller units.

Apothecary System

Apothecary weights are flat, black weights. The stamped brass dram weight, round in shape with raised characters are still used in many places. The best grain weights are aluminum wires which are less susceptible to corrosion than brass. They are more easily and quickly distinguished from each other. Aluminum weights are also more accurately adjustable than brass weight. The weight of Apothecary system in modern medicine is almost vanished. Apothecary system can be easily converted to corresponding metric system which are easier to use and less prone to errors.

Apothecary system uses the measure of unit as minim, dram (drachm) and grain for small volume measurements. For large volume measurement the units are ounces, pints, quarters, gallons and pounds. The weighing system in Apothecary system is as follows.

Fluid Measurement

1 fluid dram (drachm)	=	60 minims		
1 fluid ounce	=	8 fluid drams	=	480 minims
20 fluid ounce (fl oz)	=	1 pint		
40 fluid ounce	=	1 quarts	=	2 pints
4 quarts (160 fl oz)	=	1 gallon	=	8 pints

Solid Measurement

20 grains	=	1 scruple		
60 grains	=	3 scruple	=	1 dram
480 grains	=	8 drams	=	1 ounce
5760 grains	=	12 ounce	=	1 pound

Avoirdupois (Imperial) System

Avoirdupois weights are made of iron, flat and circular. The series of weights forms a pyramidal pile which ranges from ½ oz to 4 lb. They sometimes made of brass or zinc also and weight can be corrected by removing or adding the lead into the depression by hammering. In pharmacy cylindrical weights known as block weights are used.

The Avoirdupois system based on British standards. These systems use the base of minims, grains, drams, ounces and pounds. They are still used in pharmacy. The only difference between Apothecary system and Avoirdupois system is that their units. As per Apothecary system 1 pound is equal to 5760 grains (12 ounces) on other hand as per Avoirdupois system 1 pound is equal to 7000 grains (16 ounces). However for both Apothecary and Avoirdupois system the weight for grains is same and common for both the systems.

7000 grains	=	16 ounce	=	1 pound
437.5 grains	=	1 ounce		

Metric System

The legalization of metric system was done in 1897, but till 1971 metric system of measurement was not used in pharmaceuticals. The old prescription was seen with the abbreviation G for grams to avoid confusion between grains abbreviated as gr and cc (cubic centimeter) equivalent to ml (milliliter). For weighing larger or too smaller quantity Apothecary or Avoirdupois system of medicine fails. Modern iron metric system of weighing is replacement for that. They are preferably hexagonal and engraved letter for weight. Set of weights made of brass are usually in the range of 10 gm to 1000 gm. For small and accurate weighing a set of 10 mg to 50 gm are also available. Now a day's electronic balance are widely used with metric system of measurement. They are single pan electronic balances working on the basis of load cells. Electronic balances have facility of taring a weight of paper, container or glassware with a single push button, which facilitates weighing directly in to the final container. These balances also have internal or external calibration facilities, much easier and quicker to use, but more expensive. The prefix, symbol, names for volume and weight measurement were too easy now using metric system. The measurement range is also large. The inter-conversion calculations are in decimal of 10 and hence convenient.

Factor	Prefix	Symbol	Volume	Weight
10^{24}	yotta	Y	Yottaliter	Yottagram
10^{21}	zetta	Z	Zettaliter	Zettagram
10^{18}	exa	E	Exaliter	Exagram
10^{15}	peta	P	Petaliter	Pentagram
10^{12}	tera	T	Teraliter	Teragram
10^{9}	giga	G	Gigaliter	Gigagram
10^{6}	mega	M	Megaliter	Megagram
10^{3}	kilo	k	Kiloliter	Kilogram
10^{2}	hecto	h	Hectoliter	Hectogram
10^{1}	deka	da	Dekaliter	Dekagram
10^{-1}	deci	d	Deciliter	Decigram
10^{-2}	centi	c	Centiliter	Centigram
10^{-3}	milli	m	Milliliter	Milligram
10^{-6}	micro	μ	Microliter	Microgram
10^{-9}	nano	n	Nanoliter	Nanogram
10^{12}	pico	p	Picoliter	Picogram
10^{-15}	femto	f	Femtoliter	Femtagram
10^{-18}	atto	a	Attoliter	Attogram
10^{-21}	zepto	z	Zeptoliter	Zeptogram
10^{-24}	yocto	y	Yoctoliter	Toctogram

The following data shows the inter-conversion of Apothecary and Avoirdupois system towards metric system of measurement and commonly used abbreviations with examples for metric measurements.

1 minim	=	0.059 milliliter
1 fluid dram	=	3.6 ml
1 fluidounce	=	29.6 ml
1 pint	=	473 ml
1 gallon	=	3790 ml
1 milliliter	=	16.9 minim
1 liter	=	35.2 fluidounce
1 grain	=	64.8 mg
1 gram	=	15.4 grains
1 ounce (Apothe)	=	31.1 gram
1 ounce (Avoird)	=	28.4 gram

1 pound (Apothe)	=	373 gram
1 pound (Avoird)	=	454 gram
1 Kilogram	=	2.20 pound (Avoird)

Abbreviation and meaning	Example
kilo (k): one thousand	kilogram (kg); drug dosing commonly needs the patient's weight in kg
deci (d): one-tenth	deciliter (dL); some drug concentrations are reported as g/dL
centi (c): one-hundredth	centimeter (cm); patient's height often has to be converted from inches to cm
milli (m): one-thousandth	milliliter (mL); most injectable drug amounts are in mL
micro (mc or μ): one-millionth	microgram (mcg or μg); some drugs have low serum concentrations, e.g., mcg/L (mcg is preferred)
nano (n):one-billionth (ng);	Nanogram; some drugs have very low serum concentrations, e.g., ng/L
pico (p):one-trillionth	picogram (pg); a few drugs have barely detectable concentrations, e.g., pg/L

Common House Hold System

The house hold system consists of bits of both Apothecary and Avoirdupois system with house hold measurement devices. The system is commonly used in United States of America. Now a day common house hold system has been replaced by metric system. House hold system is still practice where measurement devices may not be available. The volume prescribed by physician in term of Apothecary or Avoirdupois system must be understood and converted to metric system first and then metric system is converted to common house hold system by pharmacist and communicated to the patient in his language. Some common house hold conversion from empirical and metric equivalence is listed below.

House hold system		***Empirical equivalence***		***Metric equivalence***
1 drop	=	1 minim	=	0.04 ml
1 teaspoonful	=	1 fluid dram	=	4 ml
1 dessertspoonful	=	2 fluid dram	=	8 ml

1 table spoonful	=	4 fluid dram	=	15 ml
1 winglassful	=	2 fluid ounce	=	60 ml
1 teacupful	=	4 fluid ounce	=	120 ml
1 tumblerful	=	8 fluid ounce	=	240 ml

Posology

The word posology is derived from Greek work "*posos*" meaning "*how much*" and "*logos*" means "*science*". Hence posology is the science that deals with dosage of drug. It also includes study of fixing of dose, calculation of dose considering the age, condition of the patient and severity of disease. The dose of a drug is always expressed in the range. The minimum dose of a drug is the quantity of drug required to elucidate the therapeutic effect and maximum dose is the highest limit or maximum quantity of drug that can be given and tolerated by the patient. The pharmacist must know the range of dose for a particular drug for therapeutic efficacy as well as for safety of patient so that the patient can be cured from disorder without getting affected by the side effects.

Factors Influencing the Dose Selection

The actual dose of the drug depends on various factors like age, gender, body weight, disease condition, nutritional status, pathological status, tolerance, route and time of drug administration, co-administration of other drugs idiosyncrasy, allergy etc.

Age

Adults requires more dose than children due to their large surface area and body volume. Similarly geriatric patients also require less quantity of medicament as compared to adults due to decrease body mass and week metabolic status of body.

Gender

Gender of patient is important during hormonal treatment. Male has more body fat as compared to female and hence requires higher dose. Female requires smaller dose than males.

Body Weight

The dose of drug is decided upon the average body weight of 70 kg for adult. However significant high or low body weight may require change in dose as per the body weight.

Disease Condition

The dose of drug also depends on severity of the disease. For example, dose of propranolol may range from 20 mg to 200 mg per day in divided dose and depends on degree of hypertension. However any degree iron deficiency anemia requires same dose of iron salt. The degree of iron absorption remains same irrespective of severity of the disease because there is limit for absorption of iron from intestine.

Nutritional Status

A patient who is already anemic or incapacitated requires less amount of dose as compared to normal individual. The same dose will produce toxic effect in that patient. Myxedematous patients are less responsive to drugs due to depressed metabolic status.

Pathological Status

Patients having organ failure required for metabolism of excretion requires smaller dose as compared to other patient. Dose of phenobarbitone must be reduced in patients with renal insufficiency. Aspirin reduces elevated body temperature but do not have any effect in normal person.

Tolerance

Some patients tolerate comparative large dose of drug. Frequent administration of drug like morphine or cocaine requires increase in dose due to development of tolerance.

Route and Time of Drug Administration

Route of administration decides rate of absorption of drug and its bioavailability in systemic circulation. Drug if given intravenously, rapidly gets distributed in body without the phase of absorption and hence comparative low dose is required. In asthmatic patient oral dose of salbutamol is around 2 mg however if given by inhalation 100 microgram is the prescribed dose. Sedatives if taken at bed time indices sleep but if taken in morning requires higher dose of drug to induce same degree of sedation.

Co-Administration of Other Drugs

Simultaneously administration of two or more drug leads to various conditions like addition, synergism or antagonism. When two or more drug given combined together give the effect equal to the addition of the individual effect of the drug then the phenomenon is known as addition. For example, beta blockers and thiazide produces additive effect. When two or more drug given combined together give the effect more than the addition of the individual effect of the drug then the phenomenon is known as synergism. For example, levodopa and carbidopa in treatment of parkinsonism or trimethoprim and sulfamethoxazole is a better antimicrobial when given combined together. When two or more drug given combined together give the less effect than the addition of the individual effect of the drug then the phenomenon is known as antagonism. For example, protamine reduces the anticoagulant action of heparin, histamine action can be blocked by pheneramine and ranitidine.

Idiosyncrasy

Idiosyncrasy is unusual reaction indicated by a specific patient to a drug. The reaction shown by patient is not manifest in majority of condition. But it is evidenced in specific patient. For example, morphine causes excitation although it is known to be a depressant of central nervous system.

Allergy

Allergy is the interaction of drug or its metabolite with body leading to an uncertain reactions. Administration of penicillin produces anaphylactic shock in allergic patient to it. Allergy generally produced due to production of antibodies.

Calculation of Pediatric Dose

Various formulas are used for calculation of different dosage from average adult dose. These formulas depend of age, body weight, surface area etc. Young's formula, Dilling's formula, Cowling's formula, Fried's formula, Bastedo's formula, Clark's formula depends on age of the pediatric patient. Catzel derived formula depends on body surface area.

- Young's formula $\text{Dose of child} = \frac{\text{Age in year}}{\text{Age} + 12} \times \text{adult dose}$
- Dilling's formula $\text{Dose of child} = \frac{\text{Age in year}}{20} \times \text{adult dose}$
- Cowling's formula $\text{Dose of child} = \frac{\text{Age in year} + 1}{24} \times \text{adult dose}$
- Fried's formula $\text{Dose of child} = \frac{\text{Age in month}}{150} \times \text{adult dose}$
- Bastedo's formula $\text{Dose of child} = \frac{\text{Age in year} + 3}{30} \times \text{adult dose}$
- Clark's formula $\text{Dose of child} = \frac{\text{Weight in pound}}{150} \times \text{adult dose}$
- Catzel's formula

$$\text{Dose of child} = \frac{\text{surface area of child} \times 100}{\text{surface area of adult}} \times \text{\% of adult dose}$$

OR $$\text{Dose of child} = \frac{\text{Body surface area of child}}{\text{Body surface area of adult}} \times \text{adult dose}$$

OR $$\text{Dose of child} = \frac{\text{Body surface area of child}}{1.73} \times \text{adult dose}$$

Latin Terms

Prescriptions written in illegible handwriting are difficult to understand by pharmacist. Use of Latin abbreviations may add mysterious appearance but ease to pharmacist to understand the prescription. For patients prescription with Latin terminology is mystery. Many countries like UK discourage prescription writing in Latin. However use of some Latin terms still persists and abbreviations are still used. Great care should be taken to avoid errors arising from misunderstanding of the Latin terms. Followings are some of Latin terms still used and helpful in current practice.

Latin term	***Abbrev.***	***English***	***Latin term***	***Abbrev.***	***English***
ad	ad.	Up to	Collunarium	collun.	Mouthwash
ad libitum	ad lib.	As much as desired	Collyrium	collyr.	Eye lotion
alternus	alt.	Alternate	compositus	Co.	Compound
ana	aa	of each	concentratus	conc.	Concentrated
ante	ante	Before	Cremor	crem.	Cream
ante cibos	a.c.	Before meal	cum	c.	With
ante cibum	a.c.	Before meal	destillatus	dest.	Distilled
ante meridiem	a.m.	Before noon	dies	d.	A day
aqua	aq.	Water	duplex	dup.	Double
aqua destillata	aq. dest.	Distilled water	ex aqua	ex aq.	In water
bis	b.	Twice	fiat	Ft., F	Make
bis die	b.d.	Twice daily	Haustus	ht.	Draught
bis in die	b.i.d.	Twice daily	hora	h.	At each hour
calidus	calid.	Warm	horasomni	h.s.	At bedtime
capiat	cap.	Take	inter cibos	i.c.	Between meal
Capsula	caps.	Capsules	Liquor	liq.	Solution
charta	chart.	Paper	mane	m.	In the morning
cibus	cib.	Food	Mistura	mist.	Mixture

Table *Contd…*

Latin term	***Abbrev.***	***English***	***Latin term***	***Abbrev.***	***English***
mitte	mitt.	Send	quaque	qq.	Every
more dicto	m.d.	As directed	quaquehora	qq.h.	Every hour
Naristillae	narist.	Nose drops	quarter die	q.d.	Four times a day
nocte	n.	At night	quarter in die	q.i.d.	Four times a day
nocte	noct.	At night	recipe	Rx	Take
nocte et mane	n. et m.	Night and morning	semisse	ss.	Half
noctemaneque	n.m.	Night and morning	si opus sit	s.o.s.	If necessary
Oculentum	oculent.	Eye ointment	signa	sig.	Label
omni die	o.d.	Every day	sine	s.	Without
omninocte	o.n.	Every night	statim	stat.	Immediately
partes	pp.	Parts	ter in die	t.i.d.	Three time a day
partiaffectae	p.a.	To the affected part	tussis	tuss	A cough
Pasta	past.	Paste	Unguentum	ung.	Ointment
per os	p.o.	Orally	ut dictum	ut. dict.	As directed
post cibum	p.c.	After meal	utantea	u.a.	As before
post meridiem	p.m.	Afternoon	utdirectum	ut.direct.	As directed
pro re nata	p.r.n.	When required	utendus	utend.	To be used
Pulvis	pulv.	Powder	Vapor	vap.	Inhalation

References

A.J. Winfield, R.M.E. Richards (2004). Pharmaceutical Practice, 3rd edition, Churchill Livingstone.

Ambler Thompson and Barry N. Taylor (2008). Guide for the use of the international system of units (SI). National Institute of Standards and technology: Special Publication 811.

B. Braun Melsungen AG (2011). Hospital Care: drug incompatibility, Risk prevention in infusion therapy, 3rd edition, from www.bbraun.com.

College of Respiratory Therapists of Ontario, Professional Practice guide, Dispensing Medications Professional Practice Guide line (2006).

Cooper and Gunn (1987). Dispensing for Pharmaceutical Students, 12th edition, CBS publishers and distributors.

Diane M. Collett, Michael E. Aulton (1996). Pharmaceutical Practice, 1st edition, Churchill Livingstone, Edinburgh London Melbourne and New York 1990.

K.G. Ravikumar, B.D. Miglani (2009). A Textbook of Pharmacy Practice, 1st edition, Career Publications.

N.K. Jain, G.D. Gupta (2009). Modern Dispensing Pharmacy, 2nd edition, PharmaMed Press, Hyderabad.

N.K. Jain, S.N. Sharma (1997). A text book of Professional Pharmacy, 4th edition, VallabhPrakashan, New Delhi.

P Jagadish Prasad (2010). Conceptial Pharmacology, 1st edition, University Press, Hyderabad.

Peter G Homan (2002). Balances, weights and measures, Information sheet 11, Royal Pharmaceutical Society.

Peter G Homan FRPharmS MCPP (2002). Chapter 3, Metric System.

Pharmaceutical Management (2012). Chapter 30: Ensuring good dispensing practice; management science for health.

Pharmacist checklist for Dispensing of controlled substances (2008). *Pharmacist checklist* **5:** 80.

Pharmacopoeial forum **35(5):** 1260 - 1310.

Pharmacy Board of Australia; Guidelines for Dispensing of medicines; from http://www.guild.org.au/qcpp/content.asp?id=807.

Ram I. Mahato (2009). Dosage Forms and Drug Delivery Systems: Apha's Complete Review for Pharmacy.

Remington (2005). The Science and Practice of Pharmacy, 21st edition, Lippincott Williams & Wilkins.

Robotic dispensing; Automation in pharmacy National Medicines Safety and Quality Scoping study report. Australian Commission on Safety and Quality in Health care. (Nov. 2010). Sydney.

Standard operating procedure for dispensing private prescriptions; from www.pharmacycpa.com.

Understanding Pharmacy calculations; Things You'll use every day.

CHAPTER 4

Hospital Pharmacy

Definition, Organization, Function and Responsibilities

A hospital is an institute or place where patients receive treatment for illness. Patients will get medical, surgical, treatment. Patient will also get the nursing care psychiatric treatment, food and lodging during course of treatment. Hospital pharmacy is the practice of pharmacy in hospital setup to cater the need of medicine for patients. It includes organizationally related facilities and services. It is department of hospital where activities related to medication are carried out which includes procurement, storage, compounding, manufacturing, packing, controlling, dispensing and distribution of medicaments. In the simple form Hospital pharmacy is defined as "portion of hospital where drugs, medicines, devices, and other materials used in the diagnosis and treatment of injury, illness and disease are dispensed, manufactured, produced, sold and distributed". All the activities are performed by a registered pharmacist who is legally qualified, professionally competent. The hospital pharmacy shop should be registered with food and drug administration and other legal authorities who issues certification from that time to time and govern these hospital pharmacy shops. In addition to these functions pharmacist is also responsible for safe and appropriate use of medication, dosing, counseling and monitoring of the patients overall therapy. The professional responsibilities are fulfilled in collaboration with other healthcare professionals. The collaboration includes development of protocol, guidelines, formularies, policies for safe use of medicines.

Organization

Uniqueness in the hospital pharmacy service is that it works in coordination with other departments of hospital which will affect the helps in effective functioning of the hospital and ultimately overall health care system. The administrators of hospital pharmacy implements the policies of governing board, delegates the authorities and passes on the responsibilities to the departmental heads, that is pharmacist in case of hospital pharmacy. The pharmacist then participates in patient's care, teaching, research activities and health related activities to achieve the objectives of the hospital. The chief pharmacist is required to coordinate all the expected services and activities delegated to the department. Pharmacist has to manage these activities in coordination with heads of other departments like finance, maintenance, security, human resource development, clinical laboratory etc. The pharmacist works in collaboration with all these departments to assure safe, efficient, and cost effective distribution and use of medicines. The accreditation agencies, licensing authorities, Food and Drug administration, regulatory authorities for standards, social and welfare agencies, the governing board and public opinion has influence on the practice of pharmacy. Because the hospital is an institute for community it is largely influenced directly or indirectly by the needs, expectations and demands of the patients and members of the community.

The hospital pharmacy is also a part of hospital administration. The ownership of this pharmacy may be an agency not concerned with the hospital and individual or may be to the hospital administration itself. When the final authority is hospital administration the chairman, team of directors, secretary of hospital governs the hospital pharmacy administration. The Director Hospital pharmacy will be in-charge of the hospital pharmacy. He is known as Director of pharmacy. The necessary licenses needed for shops are issued in the name of director of pharmacy. Director of pharmacy is responsible for all the activity in the shop including financial, legal and ethical activities. Hospital administration may acquire contractual services from registered pharmacist for the same.

The Director of pharmacy is supported and assisted by sufficient number of associate directors, assistant directors and additional pharmacist. These supporting staff may be registered (pharmacist)pharmacists or may be qualified as pharmacist (but not registered and having sufficient qualification and experience). The number of associate director, assistant directors and assisted pharmacist may be any number depending upon the workload of pharmacy. The non-registered pharmacist can work as ancillary person and should not do any work or task in which a registered pharmacist is must as per the legal requirement like manufacturing, dispensing, counseling, billing etc. These ancillary staff will assist the registered pharmacist in performing their jobs and tasks. These supporting directors, pharmacist and ancillary staff should be approved by the director of pharmacist. The director of pharmacy should develop and implement a policy and procedure to specify the duties of such supporting approved pharmacist and ancillary staff and also of any other technical person appointed if any like computer operator, peon, housekeeping persons etc. The policies and procedures should be well defined for supporting staff to avoid any accidental act which will lead to illegal activity, procedure or operation in the hospital pharmacy. The Director of pharmacy should monitor and avoid such activities and is responsible for these activities and legally will be held responsible for such activities in hospital pharmacy (figure 4.1).

Secretarial support may also be provided to the director of pharmacy for assisting his work like record keeping, report submissions, financial management and other administrative task. The secretarial staff should not do any act described for registered pharmacy as a legal obligation. All the activities and operations in the hospital pharmacy must be personally and directly supervised by director of pharmacy. All the functions and activities of other registered pharmacists and other ancillary staff should be monitored for effective, competitive, safe and without risk activities towards patient's care.

During the time when the Director of pharmacist is absent, the hospital pharmacy should not be operated unattended by any other associate/assistant director or pharmacist or other persons. The alternate arrangement must be made in advance by the director of pharmacy by appointing or authorizing the other competitive, qualified and registered pharmacist. His name must be informed and approved from legal authorities for the same.

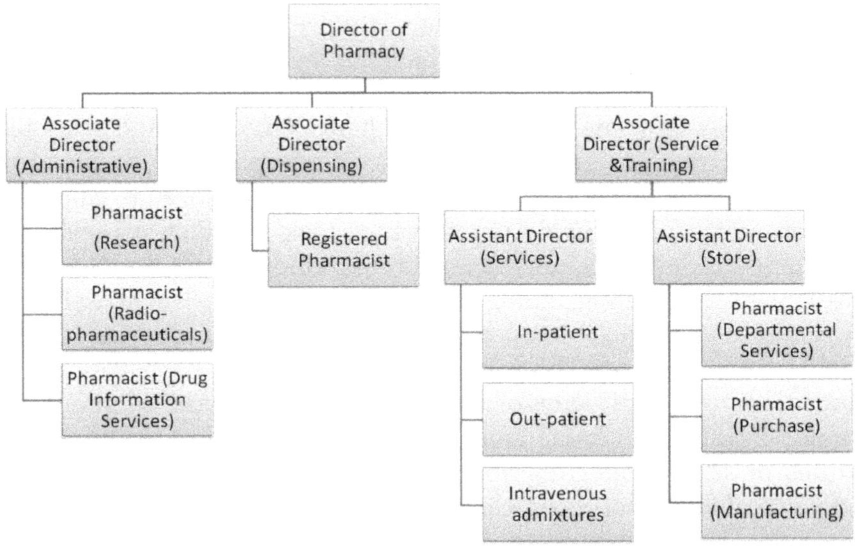

Fig. 4.1 Organization of hospital pharmacy

Functions and Responsibilities

The functions of Hospital pharmacy were outlined and approved by the American Hospital Association (AHA). It states that the department of pharmacy carries out its functions according to the philosophy and objectives of the hospital. The governing board establishes the philosophy and objective of the hospital, and accordingly pharmacist reports to the administrator of the hospital. Within the framework of hospital pharmacy it is the responsibility of pharmacist to develop high quality pharmaceutical services and in turns health services to the community. These services are for diagnostic, therapeutic, nursing and for hospital medical staff and intern's hospital as a whole.

The functions of hospital pharmacy are:

- To prepare, modify and publish hospital formulary and news bulletins in hospital.
- To make policies, take decisions, put recommendations and suggestions to pharmacy and therapeutic committee of hospital.
- Procurement, storage, compounding, dispensing, distribution and inventory control of the drugs, medicaments and other appliances for patients and hospital use.

- To provide services for medical care to the patients in fulfillment of the objectives and policies of the hospital.
- To implement services for the philosophy of hospital and to achieve objectives and standards of the hospital.
- To prepare and implement the plan for departmental administration and to define and implement the roles and responsibilities of the staff in the department.
- Coordination with other department and participation in coordinated activities in fulfillment of the services provided by the hospitals.
- To analyze and estimate the requirement of the department and to recommend and implement the policies and procedures for maintenance of adequate and competent staff.
- To provide means and methods for working in collaboration with other groups in fulfillment of the objectives of the hospitals and department in relation to patients care and community service.
- To develop and implement the system for effective maintenance of administrative and clinical record.
- To participate in the clinical trial activity (if any) and data recording and data maintenance thereof.
- To analyze the need, make necessary arrangements for supply for the facilities, equipments along with implementation of such systems, evaluation, control and maintenance.
- To establish, run and periodic update of the Medicine Information Centre in the hospital.
- Adherence to the financial plans and operations of the hospital and work in the area of limit of financial authorities and constrains provided by hospital administration.
- To participate, utilize and initiate the studies and research activities for the improvement in the patient's care and hospital services.
- To prepare and implement continuous education programs for the staff of the hospital.
- To participate and to facilitate the programs for students experience in the department.
- To organize, participate and maintain the safety procedures and equipments in the hospital.

- To organize and implement safety programs, training, demonstrations in the hospital.
- To do all the means for better patient care and hospital service in ethical and legal manner.

The hospital pharmacy involvement in health care system includes two types of relationships. The one type is related to the patients and other related to the medicine procurement. The hospital pharmacy has to keep pace with laboratory, laboratory data and supply of laboratory needs. In total terns it deals with patient's care. It should also be in tune with facility department and financial department which will take care of financial aspects of patient's treatment cost.

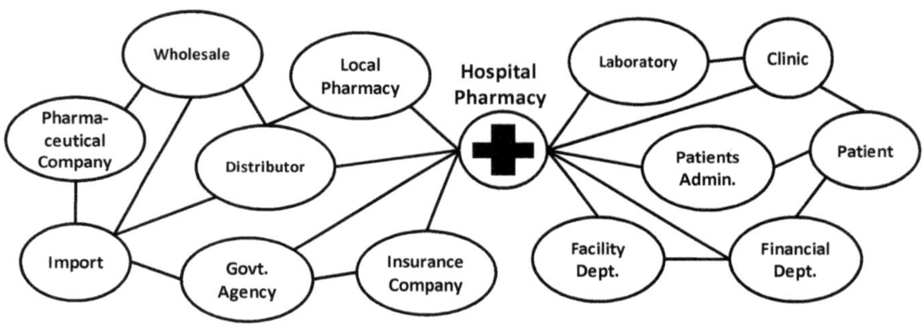

Fig. 4.2 Agencies dealing with hospital pharmacy

The hospital pharmacy also deals with various agencies involved in medicine procurement like distributors, Govt. agencies, local pharmacies, insurance companies, importers, pharmaceutical companies, and wholesalers. This aspect of hospital pharmacy is not having any direct relation with patient's care but the ultimate outcome is related to patient's care only. The medicines procured by all the means will be used for patient's treatment and care. The hospital pharmacy act as a interface between various external medicine stakeholders and agencies involved in supply of medicines *(left side of the figure)* and the various internal departments of hospitals involving patients, clinicians, laboratory etc. *(right side of the figure)*. For instance, the hospital pharmacy is not only responsible for drugs supply but also offers consultancy services to clinics, prepares and supply of medical devices for the laboratory, provides additional information for the patient administration department, the financial department, patient counseling, procurement of medicines, drugs and equipments from external agencies etc.

Health Care System

Health care is huge number of services given to individual, his family, group of peoples or community by the agency of health service for purpose of promoting, maintaining, monitoring or restoring the health. The system which renders these services is health care system. These services that health care system provides to the patients by the health care professionals include diagnosis, care, help, education, counseling, advice, rehabilitation etc. Prescribing the medicines, dispensing, administration of drugs are the personal services while health care system is a social service. Depending on the nature (evolution) of illness, injury and nature of treatment the scope of hospitals, services rendered and organization itself are changing. The major factor contributing in this evolution is advances in medicine, technology and changing needs and expectation of the patients. The advertisement in medicine and technology allows the patients to care for it requirements like nature of intensive care unit, ambulatory services, skilled nursing staff etc. As a result of which the patients are getting good medical care. The development of ambulatory surgery centers, home health services, outpatient treatment centers and multiple disease monitoring facilities are the outcomes evidenced for development in health care services. Health care services are continuously searching to meet the need of patients demand for safe, quality health care with affordable cost. This mission leads to a development of better hospitals for better health care system and services like primary care, outpatient care, home care, nursing facility and also includes health insurance schemes.

In earlier days the role of hospital pharmacy was limited to distribution of medicine. Hospital pharmacy travelled a long journey from counting, licking and pouring related to the medicine to become a full-fledged hospital pharmacy as a department. Now days in hospitals, the hospital pharmacy is not only a simple medicine ordering and filling carts. They are heavily involved in all aspects of patients care. Number of clinical responsibilities has lead to the impact on patient's health. It was observed that interaction of healthcare team during patients round, interviewing patients, reconciling medicine and providing patients counseling during discharge result in significant reduction in adverse drug events, medication errors, length of stay and thus leading to improvement in medical adherence.

The role of hospital pharmacist is changing as per the new emerging concept of pharmaceutical care. The role of pharmacist is changing from traditional medicine oriented dispensing to patient centered practice model. In this practice pharmacist assure the responsibility for therapeutic outcome of medicine and improves the patients adherence and use the medicine related experience and expertise for batter patients care. The hospital pharmacist assists the patient by educating the patient about the disorder and need of timely medicine, monitoring the patient's medication, increasing the collaboration of prescribing clinician and by that way avoids the errors in prescriptions and other problems like drug - drug, drug - food interactions, etc.

India's health care system spends lowest amongst worldwide. It's around US$ 4 per person per year as compare to around US$ 2000 per person per year in United States. Indian system has sharply increased their spending on health care system from 1990's. As per government setup the Indian health care system is categorized in three levels - primary, secondary and tertiary. Primary health care system includes PHC (primary health centers) that is the first contact between patient and health care professionals. Some health related problems can be solved at PHC level with cheapest cost. India has a wast network of PHC and serves for billion peoples with ratio of around 1 clinic for 3000 to 5000 peoples. PHC are present almost in every taluka level in India. Secondary health care centers are extensions of PHC. Patients are referred from PHC to secondary health care centers where more complicated health problems are handled. Secondary health care centers are present at taluka and district level. District hospitals come under the category of secondary health care center. The tertiary health care hospitals are present at regional or state level and provide specialty or super-specialty facilities for health care system. They provide highest level of specialization and also teaching facilities and provide facilities of training for specialized staff. The Civil hospitals are denoted as tertiary hospitals. Along with the network of government hospitals the private, co-operative and military hospitals also cater the need of health care system. Many private organizations, NGO's and government organizations also run the large number of hospitals.

Hospital Drug Policy

Before 1950s very few drug molecules were available for the treatment of diseases like analgesic and antipyretics (aspirin and morphine), antimalarial (quinine), cardiovascular drug (digitalis) etc. The development in pharmaceutical and medicinal chemistry introduces a large number of chemicals in therapeutics drugs with very high potency, broad spectrum of activity. Introduction of these new molecules creates a problem in selection of appropriate drug molecule for the treatment. Low therapeutic index due to high potency, development of resistance and tolerance cannot be overlooked especially for antimicrobial agents. When a large number of drugs are available for the treatment in the same area of diseases, the selection of appropriate drug by considering patient's history, nature of disease, frequency of drug administration requires guidelines for the physician. These guidelines to be provided by hospital administration will help the medical professionals for selection of drug in treatment. In fulfilling these objectives and need, the concept of Pharmacy and therapeutic committee (PTC), Drug and therapeutic committee (DTC) came into existence. Many hospitals has developed the PTC/DTC, hospital formulary, hospital committees, therapeutic guidelines and newsletters for better healthcare facilities

PTC

Pharmacy and therapeutic committee (PTC) is also known as pharmacy committee, drug committee or drug and therapeutic committee (DTC). The drug and therapeutic committee is essential component of health care system for selection of medicine, distribution and use. PTC has many functions related to selection and rational use of medicaments. PTC develops policies for managing pharmaceutical use, administration and formulary system in the hospital. This committee is dedicated to prepare and maintenance of list of medicines for hospital and clinical usage. PTC is policy recommending body and not policy implementing body. It can recommend, suggest but cannot make it compulsory to the medical practitioner to strict implement that policy. Physician has freedom to use the drugs against policy in special cases. PTC is tool for self-restriction and control on rational and ethical use of drugs. The PTC has number of responsibilities and performed successfully. Its function has positive impact on patient's health care.

No single person can have a detail knowledge of a drug and knowledge of all the drugs from different categories. This is the main motto behind constitution of PTC in the hospitals. The composition and constitution of PTC depends of the function, nature, type of hospital and the activities carried out in the hospital. The American Hospital Association and American Society of Hospital Pharmacists suggest that PTC should compose of minimum three physicians, one pharmacist, one nurse, authorities of hospital administration etc. The pharmacist is designated as secretary. The agenda of meeting and other necessary document should be prepared by the secretary and send to the members of committee well in advance for the study. The minutes of meeting should be prepared by the secretary and maintain record of it. The recommendations of PTC should be presented before appropriate committee for approval and the action of such committee should be communicated to various health care persons who will implement it. The PTC should have meeting regularly at least once a month or not less than twice per year. They also should meet on call when necessary and requires opinion in special circumstances. The PTC should constitute various members as follows.

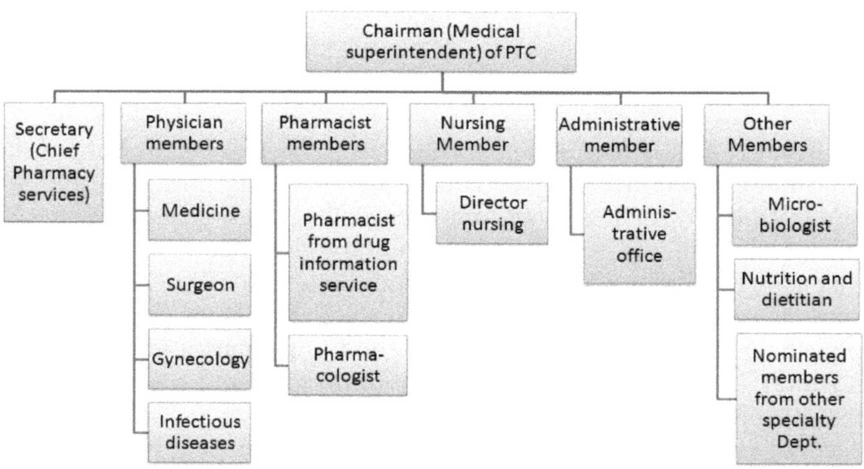

When specific issues are to be handled like introduction of newly discovered medicines or related issues then PTC may invite specialist in the meeting. This member can be outside the PTC or even outside the hospital and a specialist or expert in the concerned field. Such invited expert does not have voting privilege. But such expert gives advice on such issues. Accepting or rejecting his opinion depends on the PTC. To perform a specific task PTC may form a subcommittee. This subcommittee has a limited life span up to the completion of task. Some authorities and responsibilities will be dedicated to this committee for effective functioning and such subcommittees can have their (out) own meetings for effective completion of tasks. The performance of such subcommittees will be monitored by PTC.

For effective functioning of PTC certain principles must be framed and adopted. These functions are followed throughout the activity of committee and during committee proceedings. The principles include transparency and unbiased decisions, clear objectives and evidence based approach, consistency in activity, impact oriented attitude etc. Following factors are involved in the effective and long lasting functioning of PTC

- Establishment of clear goals and functions of PTC.
- Wide representation in the constitution of PTC.
- No permission in PTC to the owner or relative of pharmaceutical or other manufacturer or supplier.
- The committee should communicate all the information, policy, procedure, recommendations and activities to all the hospital staff without hiding the matter or part of it.
- PTC should obtain official status by taking appropriate permission from hospital administration.
- Should ensure that committee is motivated and actively participating in decision making.
- It should support the medical and pharmacy department and to other social activities of the hospital.
- PTC should ensure payment of appropriate incentives to the committee members and performers in the hospital.

The committee must operate in a manner that confirms the transparency and it should avoid conflicts of interest with manufacturers or distributors of pharmaceuticals and suppliers of medical appliances. A strict ethical policy should be developed and rigidly enforced at all the time for maintaining objectivity and credibility. The committee or its any member should not have any relationship with pharmaceutical companies, supplier other than a purely professional official person that will encourages the acquisition of quality medicines to the hospital and the flow of unbiased information about their products to the staff of the hospital.

The function of PTC and acquired benefits and advantages includes:

- Selection of effective, high quality, safe and cost effective drug for treatment.
- Advice the medical staff in matters related to drug usage. The PTC is a valuable asset for medical staff, administration, pharmacy and other hospital department in organizing the health care system. The committee provides recommendations and advisory service in aspects of the drug.
- To frame and recommend the policy regarding safe use of drug in hospital.
- Development and implementation of guidelines for generic drug policy and therapeutic substitution policy.
- Locating the problem related to use of medicine and improvement in it suggesting alternate medicines.
- Advice the medical staff for selection of drugs and choice of drugs available to meet the effective therapy.
- To recommend the measures in prevention of duplication of drug usage.
- Framing, recommendation and adaptation of suitable policy, evaluate problem related to selection, procurement, storage, prescribing, dispensing and usage of medicine. PTC is responsible for development of pharmaceutical policy in the health organization necessary for adequate control of medicine selection, purchase, distribution, use and administration.
- Advice the management, regulating policy framing and implementation for issues related to use of investigational drugs in hospital.
- PTC evaluates and selects medicines to be incorporated in the formulary. Evaluating medicine and consequently approving or rejecting it before incorporation in the formulary taking in account the expertise opinion is the function of PTC.
- To manage the clinical data regarding new drugs.

- Improvement in medicinal value through rational utilization and quality of patient's health and outcomes.
- Management of resistance developed by the medicine especially antimicrobial agents.
- To assist in designing the framework, policy, planning for education and content updating programs regarding matters related to drug and their use.
- To define the procedure, framing policy and steps for development, modification, amendment in the hospital formulary.
- Increased staff knowledge by continuing education programs and also patient's knowledge by counseling.
- Effective monitoring and taking measures for management of adverse drug reactions and medication errors.
- Monitoring discharges patients for long term use of drug.
- Effective management and improving in medicine inventory.
- Managing and control of expenditure of treatment and pharmaceuticals.

Hospital Formulary

Hospital formulary is official listing or book of drugs approved by committees in the hospital for use in hospitals. The purpose of hospital formulary is to ensure the availability of safe, therapeutically and cost effective medications to the patients. Hospital formulary is continuously update list and related information of the drug. Updating involves clinical judgments of physician, pharmacist and other experts in the field of diagnosis, treatment of disease and health promotions. Hospital formulary system is the continuous ongoing process by which health care professionals establishes policy on the use of drug and products that will be medically most appropriate, cost effective and provide best treatment in the interest of patient. PTC is the advisory committee responsible for defining the policies of hospital pharmacy. PTC is also involved in development, management, updating and administrating the hospital formulary.

PTC is responsible for incorporation of the name of drug and its detail in the hospital formulary. The clinical decisions are based on the scientific evidences and standard practice in the clinic. It does not include the facts and findings that are from peer-reviewed medical literature, random clinical trials, pharmacoeconomic studies or outcome of some research data. The decision of incorporation of name of drug is based on practice guidelines and documents developed by acceptable evidence based facts, comparison of efficacy, type and frequency of side effect and potential drug interaction, effect of drug on patient's compliance as compared to other products. The economic consideration should be taken in to account during formulary development which include:

- Decision on cost factor after establishment of safety
- Efficacy and therapeutic need
- Evaluation of drug on the basis of impact on total health care cost
- Financial benefit on the basis of cost management and not on the basis of drug therapeutics

The formulary system should provide drug product selection and formulary maintenance. It provides method of evaluation and periodic analysis of drug used for maintenance and enhancement of quality of patients care by assured drug treatment. It also provides means for monitoring, reporting and analysis of adverse reactions of drug therapy. The system inform the clinical practitioners about the modification and decisions in hospital formulary that will ensure cost reduction in treatment, better therapeutically effective and safe drug and procedure for obtaining the non-formulary drugs. It also informs the changes took place in formulary. The formulary system provides patient's education programs, measures for improvement in the patient's compliance and adherence. System takes measure for easy availability and accessibility of the hospital formulary. The hospital formulary system also ensure that the patient will get a non-formulary drug when clinically justified by the physician and make a provision to that effect in formulary itself. The system also develops a process for timely procurement of such non-formulary drugs. It should have minimal and well define approval process obtaining non-formulary drug and should have a process of appeal if request is denied. The system should not panelize the practitioner for asking the non-formulary drug if justified the medical need.

The hospital formulary has its own disadvantages and limitations. The hospital formulary system deprives the physician from his right of selection of drugs, freedom for prescription and obtaining a brand of his choice. Hospital formulary system gives whole authority to the pharmacist to purchase and obtain the brand of drug and dispense. The system may procure the large quantity of drug to reduce the cost of the drug but this reduced cost may not be passed to the patients and patients has to purchase a drug at elevated cost even though a substitute may be available at comparative low cost.

For the development and maintenance of formulary and formulary system in hospital different approaches can be used. The single formulary can be developed for a group of facilities and clinicians. The steps involved in hospital formulary development include:

Administrative

- Concept introduction and taking support from administration
- Establishment of committee
- Deciding and development of policies and procedures

Formulary development

- Choose and develop a therapeutic classification scheme for formulary
- Data collection and analysis of existing drug usage pattern
- Analysis of morbidity and drug utilization pattern
- Conductance of drug class review
- Getting approval list for use in health care system
- Educate the staff involved in health care system for effective use of formulary

Development of formulary manual

- Decision on drug formulary and formulary manual
- Development of policy and information section
- Development of monograph for manual
- Development of information section
- Development of index
- Reproduce and distribution of manual

Formulary maintenance

- Development of standard guideline for maintenance
- Design the policy and procedure for drug use evaluation program

- Design and implement adverse drug monitoring and evaluation process
- Design the policy and implement it for updating the formulary and manual

The hospital formulary contains drug information in the following manner

1. ***Formulary list:*** Alphabetic list of medicines included in hospital formulary. Therapeutic list is also provided along with alphabetic list of drugs.
2. ***Brief information:*** This comprises of brief information about each drug and medicine including generic name, brand name, dosage form and strengths available, administration indications, contraindication and percussion, side effects, dosage schedule, instructions and warnings, drug, food and laboratory interactions.
3. ***Supplementary information:*** Comprises of price, regulatory category like schedule H drug or schedule X drug, storage guidelines like store in cool and dry place, patients counseling information, labeling information, brand name and synonyms etc.
4. ***Prescription and dispensing guidelines:*** The section give information about rational prescribing techniques, principles of prescription writing, guidelines for quantity to be dispensed, controlled drug requirement, adverse drug reporting requirement, dispensing guidelines, list of precautionary labels, common drug interaction to be monitored in description of table form etc.
5. ***Treatment protocol:*** Includes drug administration guidelines, drugs usage in pregnancy and lactating mother, drug usage in renal complications, poisoning and intoxication guidelines, pediatric and geriatric prescribing.
6. ***Other components:*** This section includes information regarding metric measurements and table, format for reporting of adverse drug reaction if found any, formulary requisition form, indices and list of abbreviation.

Hospital Committee

Other than PTC various modern hospitals also constitutes various other committees which look after and performs various function. These committees help in hospital administration and management for monitoring and controlling various activities in the hospital through framing various policies, norms and defining objectives. These all committees are associated with PTC. In various hospitals the PTC itself is given the roles and responsibilities of all these committees. Such various committees framed includes:

- **Antibiotic committee:** Antibiotics and antimicrobials are the most widely and largely used drugs in the hospital. This committee frames the guidelines, norms and policies for the use of antibiotics in the hospital so that rational use of antibiotic will be there without developing of a resistance.
- **Ethical committee:** This committee looks after the ethical issues related to the research activity carried out in the hospital.
- **Formulary committee:** This committee is dedicated to the selection of drug for incorporation into the formulary. It also includes development, maintenance, addition and deletion of the drugs from formulary time to time and as per the requirement.
- **Drug exchange and donation committee:** This committee monitors the exchange program of the drugs with other hospitals or agency. It also monitors the free distribution or donation of drugs and appliances in hospital or during camps as a charitable activity of the hospital.
- **Infection control committee:** This committee monitors the occurrence, spreading and control of the infections in various departments of the hospitals like operation theater, ICU, critical care unit etc.
- **Hospital review committee:** This committee comprises of qualified mental health professionals. Committee reviews the appropriateness of patient's treatment plan.
- **Institutional animal ethical committee:** This committee looks after the ethical and legal issues of the research activity in the hospital related to the animal experimentations.

Therapeutic guidelines: A hospital develops a drug policy to seek control on both demand and supply of drug. The hospital drug policy avoids the unnecessary criminalization of products, trafficking and use. Every attempt must be made to supply medicine to the patients in fair manner. Therapeutic guidelines describe about the various way for substitution, alteration in the drug if one drug, dosage form is not available. These substituted drugs or alteration does not compromise the therapeutic efficacy of the prescribed drug. The ways by which such substitutions and alterations permitted are as follows. Therapeutic guidelines help the pharmacist in dispensing the substituted or alternate medication of formulation in order to get better therapeutic efficacy, reduce the cost of the treatment.

Generic substitution: The generic substitution of drug products contains the same active ingredient(s) available as that of branded product. The quantity and quality of the medicament in generic product are chemically identical in strength, concentration. The dosage form is also of same kind when generic is compared with branded and route of administration to the drug product prescribed is also same. Generic substitution may or may not require permission from prescriber and seeking such permission may be a policy of the particular hospital. For e.g., chloroquine, nifedipine, codeine sustained release, ciprofloxacin/dexamethasone, clotrimazole topical, piroxicam 10/20 mg capsules, piroxicam 10/20 mg suppositories, omeprazole 20 mg, cyclosporine.

Therapeutic alternates: In the therapeutic alternate the dosage form may be same but have different chemical structures. This different chemical medicament should have same pharmacological and/or therapeutic class, and mostly expected to have similar therapeutic effects and adverse reaction profiles. When such therapeutic alternative is given they are generally administered in therapeutically equivalent doses. To dispense a therapeutic alternate drug a strict permission is needed from prescriber without which such alternate drug should not be dispensed.

Therapeutic interchange: Therapeutic interchange is authorized exchange of therapeutic alternates. This type of interchange is according to previously established and approved written guidelines or protocols within a formulary system and restricted to the jurisdiction of the hospital only.

Therapeutic substitution: The act of therapeutic substitution is similar to that of therapeutic alternate. They can be used synonymously for each other. The act of such dispensing a therapeutic alternate or substitutions for the drug product prescribed without prior authorization of the prescriber is an illegal act because only the prescriber may authorize an exchange of therapeutic alternates.

Drug Utilization Review (DUR): (Drug Use Review, DUR, and Drug Use Evaluation) this process is used to assess the appropriateness of drug therapy prescribed by the medical practitioner. The appropriateness may be checked by evaluation of data on drug use in a given health care environment against predetermined criteria and standards.

Therapeutic equivalents: The therapeutic equivalency in the different dosage form is the similarity in therapeutic benefit along with efficacy, safety, tolerance etc. These two products may have different chemical moiety from same therapeutic class in different quantity. The Pharmacy and Therapeutics Committee has to approve Therapeutic Interchange Policies in hospital formulary system. Pharmacists may be permitted to substitute a product from the same class of drug, even though they are not therapeutically equivalent. Such substitutions are permitted with or without prior permission of prescriber as per the policy decision of the hospital PTC. Therapeutic interchange is the practice of switching or dispensing drugs that are chemically distinct but therapeutically similar in terms of their efficacy, safety, and tolerability profiles. The ultimate goal of therapeutic interchange is to achieve an improved or neutral outcome with the new agent while reducing overall treatment costs.

Newsletter: A newsletter can be a valuable document published by hospital administration in providing drug information to all personals involved in health care profession. These newsletters can be published with any frequency as per the scope and need of the hospital. It can be weekly, monthly, quarterly or at longer intervals. The newsletter should provide all staff with unbiased and accurate information about drug therapy, new development and any observations reported in hospitals. Newsletters should also publish news regarding special achievements, awards, prizes, scholarships etc., of the staff. Newsletters have an advantage over group presentations that busy practitioners can read them at a time that suits them. However printed materials like newsletters are unlikely to be effective in changing irrational prescribing habits unless they are combined with a more interactive method. Newsletters are already published and distributed by commercial ventures. However a local bulletin can be an invaluable asset for hospital, since it will provide more information concerning medicines and medicine-related problems of specific interest at the local level. Newsletters are more likely to be effective in improving rational drug use if certain principles are adhered.

Principles of effective drug newsletters:

- The prescribing behavior and reasons behind them can be understood and addressed, for example, lack of knowledge, generic drug and branded drug etc.
- Availability of concise and up-to-date information of immediate use.
- Information provided in newsletter is limited and key points are repeated in boxes and highlights. Lengthy presentations of new information and reviews may lose the interest of most readers and may lose the available information.
- Short headings, visually appealing illustrations, boxes, highlights are used, so catching the attention of readers.
- The text must be brief and in simple language.
- The information presented must be obtained and derived from reputable journals and the references and cross references must be provided.
- The information provided in the newsletter must be orientated towards actions and decisions to be taken during therapy.
- Feedback from experience, expert, professional staff or even from outside expertise on the value of the newsletter is asked for and changes should be made as necessary.
- Local experts from outside hospital, institution are asked to write and comment in order to improve acceptability and credibility.
- The views, comments etc., put in newsletter should be unbiased and should not harm to the moral of any one. It should not disclose the confidential information. If necessary alternate name must be used to represent the care related to the patient.

Hospital Pharmacy Services

American pharmacist association describes a broad range of health care services provided by the pharmacists. It works as an expert on health care team. The pharmacist provides help to patients to get the best benefit from the medications they take by actively managing drug therapy and identifying and resolving drug and treatment related problems. The service they provide is in conjugation with medication. The pharmacist take care that the right medicine for the right patient to get best possible outcome for the treatment. The services provided by hospital pharmacy can be summarized as:

- **Finance:** The financial service is joint responsibility of hospital pharmacy and hospital administration. It is the National Health Policy of India that every citizen should get the medicine at affordable cost. In order to meet the gap between purchasing cost and affordable cost by the patient, various policies are to be framed by the hospital administration or a suitable financial alternative has to be found out who will take care of financial burdens of treatment cost. Government agencies, health care insurance policy, donations from non-government organization and other agencies also contribute for financial aspects.
- **Procurement:** The objective of procurement is to ensure and maintain a proper supply of medicines at best possible price. The suitable policy and procedure should be framed for procurement of medicines. Price negotiation for procurement of essential drugs and medicines supply will be undertaken by pharmacist. For the best possible price, drugs should be ordered in bulk packs and from local distributors, regional distributors or if possible directly from company warehouse. Company normally does not entertain the direct procurement of drugs from their warehouse and have their own network for sale and distribution of drugs. But as a social obligation and to reduce the cost, some companies distribute the drugs directly to the hospital where a large quantity of drugs are required. The procurement procedure should be done by publication of tenders and placing the orders to suppliers having optimal cost with high quality medicine. The tender should be issued as per public sector tender system. The high security computerized tender system has been introduced (e-tendering) which maintains the confidentiality as well as the monitors the dates,

specifications and other aspects of tendering procedures. Independent system is established which will monitor suppliers performance. The information provided by such system will be used for identification of new drug suppliers and making new contracts. The procurement will be aimed to purchase medicine with lowest available price and defined specification for quality. A bulk purchasing or even batch purchasing is done in case of chain hospitals where a large quantity will reduce the price drastically. A fast track registration procedure should be established for such kind of purchase procedures. Calling the tender for generic name of drugs, asking for patient's ready pack, preferring the drug with labelled generic solely are some of the tips which assist the procurement procedure. The tender calling and awarding should be completely transparent process to avoid any conflicts and a special tender board should be established for the same to look after it.

- **Inventory:** The objective of inventory is to maintain the quality and security of procured medicaments and other appliances in store from its time of receipt in stock till issue to the patients. Assistant will be appointed to the pharmacist to assist this kind of work which includes a formation of standard operating procedure and practical guidelines for record keeping and storage of goods. This also includes administrative procedures for management and effective control, storage and distribution, defining minimal and maximum stock levels, guidelines for stock rotation, and handling of expiry of stock and obsolete stock of drugs and medical supplies. These standard operating procedures will be used for training and supervision of staff and updating the information. Appropriate staffing and allocation of authorities and responsibilities should be done for this work. The information obtained from monitoring system will be used for determination of quantity to be procured. Effective and standard security system must be established in warehouse to monitor the material and man's trafficking.
- **Distribution:** The objective is prompt, timely and effective distribution of requirement as per need and demand to the health care practitioner and patients. Provision should be made for own distribution system and pharmacist should not

depend on the distribution system which is not under his control. Handing over the box of containers to the relatives of patients or nursing staff can be a preferred distribution network which assures the timely and accurate distribution of the drugs to the right patients. Computerized inventory control and labeling mechanism will help in timely, accurately and errorless distribution and this system also help in inventory control and stock verification. A private courier services can be hired for distribution and supply of medicine to the patients with chronic illness, referred patients, age old outpatients and during camps. The distribution of cold storage items like vaccines should be done with caution and appropriate devices like thermos box, cold storage box must be used during their transport from warehouse, refrigerator to ward or injection tables. Long term exposure of such medicament to the atmospheric temperature will deteriorate their quality and reduces efficacy.

- **Disposal:** The objective of disposal is to ensure that all the drugs, medicaments, appliances and associated waste were disposed promptly as per procedure effectively and safely. The disposal procedure and guidelines must be framed for the same and procedures must be executed in presence of appropriate authorities. A pharmacist looks after for formation and execution of method for the removal, disposal and return stock of drugs, medical supplies and medical wastes. A legislation committee should be constituted for such removal and disposal in such a manner that neither harmful nor dangerous to the community or environment. In no case the expired or nearly expired drugs, medicaments or appliances be dispensed, distributed or supplied to the patients. Authority must inspect to ensure the storage area, warehouse for labeling, isolation, removal of such stock from dispensing area as per legal and standard guidelines.

Hospital Manufacturing

Pharmacy and therapeutic committee (PTC) is formulated for preparation, updating of the hospital formulary. Hospital formulary is the list of drugs preferred for the administration in the hospital. Hospital formulary also gives the other detail information about such drugs. Consumption of some drugs from list of hospital formulary may not be significant and such drugs are procured directly from market. However some drugs like antibiotics, antibacterial are widely used in hospital and their requirement is very high. In such conditions instead of procuring these medicaments from market, hospital administration may take decision to manufacture such medicaments in hospital itself for their own use. Such hospital manufactured drugs and pharmaceuticals are exclusively for the hospital use and not for distribution to other hospitals or commercial sale outside hospital. These formulations will be manufactured in the facilities available in manufacturing plant of hospital and dispensed in hospital pharmacy. A small scale unit suitable to meet the requirement of hospital shall be established for such manufacturing.

Manufacturing in hospital must be done under the supervision of qualified and approved pharmacist as per the guidelines of Food and Drug Administration (FDA). The approved pharmacist is responsible for all the activities in such manufacturing area. The hospital administration shall decide which formulation must be manufactured at hospital level and appropriate license should be obtained from FDA for manufacturing of such formulation. The formula for such manufacturing process must be listed in hospital formulary and this formula along with manufacturing process also should be approved from FDA. All the facilities required for manufacturing of the formulation should be as per the rules and guidelines mentioned in schedule M of the FDA. All the equipments, instruments and accessory facilities must be of appropriate standards to maintain quality of the formulation. A separate quality control laboratory must be established containing all relevant facilities for quality control and analysis of raw material, in process and finished product quality control and quality analysis. The labeling of such formulations manufactured in hospital should meet the requirement of FDA. The label of such formulation will be different from labels of containers used for dispensing in hospital.

The facilities and equipments required for manufacturing in hospital are listed below. At present in India we will find such type of Pharmacy in Vellore Hospital (T.N) and Jaslok Hospital Mumbai (Maharashtra).

- **External preparations:** Equipments for manufacturing of external preparations like ointments, emulsions, lotions, solutions, pastes and creams includes mixing tanks, steam or electrically heated kettles, mechanical mixers, storage tanks, colloidal mills, triple roller mills, liquid filling machines etc.

- **Oral preparations:** Oral preparations like syrups, solutions, elixirs, emulsions, suspensions required facilities such as mixing and storage tanks, portable mixers, water stills, colloidal mills, filter press, vacuum filters, bottle filling machines, cap sealing machines etc.
- **Solid preparations:** The solid preparations include compressed tablets, pills powders etc. the facilities required includes different section which comprises of granulating section, tablet section. Granulation section requires disintegrator, granulator, mass mixer, powder mixer etc. Tablet section requires tablet machine, pill machine, punch and dies storage unit, tablet counter, tablet inspection belt, equipment for in process quality control like hardness tester, weighing balance etc., and coating equipments like jacketed kettles, coating pans, polishing pans etc. Powder manufacturing facilities include disintegrators, mixers, sifters, stainless steel vessels, filling equipments.
- **Sterile products:** Manufacturing of sterile product requires special facilities. The products like small volume and large volume parenterals, eye ointments and lotions, surgical dressing and absorbent cotton are included in sterile product manufacturing. The facilities required for such manufacturing includes hot air ovens, heating kettles, colloidal mills, mixing and storing tanks, filtering equipments, liquid filling machines etc. For preparation of sterile parenteral special aseptic manufacturing and filling area is must along with sterilization facility.

Quality control laboratory: The quality control laboratory should include all the necessary equipments required for in process and finished product analysis. The general facility includes suitable calibrated glassware, laboratory apparatus and standard grade chemicals.

Radiopharmaceuticals

Radiopharmaceuticals are used in medical profession for diagnosis and treatment of diseases. It may be a great source of man-made radiation exposure. The procurement, storage, utilization of such radiopharmaceuticals for the diagnosis, treatment of patients requires a special licensing and facilities in the hospital. There are three types of radiations used in medicinal practice. X-ray examination, nuclear medicine and radiotherapy. X-ray and nuclear medicine are the techniques used for diagnosis of injury and illness. Bone related examinations are done using X-ray techniques. In nuclear medicine gamma rays are used for diagnosis or function of critical organs. The radiation material is administered with medicine, which is absorbed by tissue to be observed for diagnosis. The distribution of drug/gamma emitting material in the tissue is observed using gamma camera. Radiotherapy is used exclusively for treatment of malignant cancer with intention of curing disease.

Handling and Packaging

During transportation and shipment the radiopharmaceutical is packed in special packages. These packages are of three types, Industrial packaging, Type A packaging and Type B packaging. In industrial packaging low and specific activity materials are transported including radioactive hospital wastes, laboratory and power plant wastes etc. Type A packaging is used for majority of radioactive material and pharmaceutical packing and transportation. The packaging is designed to withstand all the stress during transportation under non-accidental condition. Type B packaging is used for high radioactive materials like radiographic source, nuclear reactors etc. A special kind of label must be put on these containers which are of three types. Category I (Radioactive white) label is for very low radiation (less than 5 μSv/h) on the surface of container, category II (Yellow II) label is for low radiation (less than 500 μSv/h) on the surface of container whereas category III (Yellow III) label is for radiation less than 2 μSv/h) on the surface of container.

Radiopharmaceuticals are only dispensed to the hospital supply. In no case radiopharmaceuticals are dispensed to the patients or his relatives. The radioactive drug is dispensed and carried by hospital staff or authorized person from hospital staff and carried to the area where it is directly administered to the patients. Radiopharmaceuticals are stored in a separate isolated area specially designed and constructed. The area for storage of such material should be located suitable, well-lighted, well-ventilated and having clean and sanitary surrounding. All the activity related to radiopharmaceuticals should be done in the specified area only. The area should have different sections like storage, prescription counter, dispensing area, hood space, quality control area etc. All the equipments, instruments and glassware used for radiopharmaceuticals should be separate from other pharmaceuticals. The standard reference books must be maintained in nearby area of the radiopharmaceutical dispensing and storage area. The appropriate labels and warning must be put on the walls and doors of the area. A special officer should be appointed to monitor the safe use of such radiopharmaceuticals. This office will be under direct control of hospital administration and will be responsible for safety and use of radio pharmaceuticals. The record must be kept for all activities and this must contain the list of individuals who are authorized to handle the radio pharmaceuticals. The document must contain detailed information about name of trained person for handling, location where these substances will be used, storage location, inventory of used and unused substance, details about incidences happened if any, record of purchase and distribution, safety precaution, method of removal of contamination, calibration of radio measuring device, waste disposal techniques, transport document and any other such document required by controlling or legal authorities.

Most of the time the half-life of radiopharmaceutical drug is very short and it is immediately administered after their formulation and dispensing. The storage of pre-formulated radioactive formulation is very rare. Qualified, licensed, trained pharmacists formulate the dosage form and it is issued immediately and carried to the drug administration area where the formulation is immediately administered to the patients. Storage of such formulation leads to significant loss of the radioactivity and may reduce its therapeutic value. A great care must be taken during transfer of radiopharmaceuticals from dispensing area to the administration area. Dispensing area of hospital should not be contaminated by the radioactive material. The handling of radioactive material should be done in a tray containing high absorbent tissue paper so that any spillage will be absorbed by the paper. Rubber gloves must be used during handling of the radioactive material. The mouth operated aspiration tubes or pipettes should not be used. The waste material should be stored till radio activity get minimal suitable for disposal. A great care must be taken before disposal of any kind of waste generated from area where radioactive material is handled, stored, dispensed or administered. Activities like smoking, drinking, eating are strictly prohibited in the area where radioactive material is handled. The radioactivity emitter should never be handled with hand and forceps must be used. Sufficient shielding cloths and devices must be put on before entering in the area. The radioactive material must be stored in suitable labeled container, shielded by specially made bricks and stored preferably in remote corner. A regular monitoring of the radioactivity must be done in the area where radioactive material is stored, handled, dispensed or administered.

Indian Scenario

In 1752, Jonathan Robert was claimed to be the first hospital pharmacist of Pennsylvania Hospital from colonial America. In Indian contest no such record was observed reporting emerge of hospital pharmacy filed. Significant advancement in hospital pharmacy in India took place from 1960 onwards. The credit of development goes to American Hospital Pharmacist Association and Indian Hospital Pharmacist Association.

In 1847 Madras Medical College admitted five candidates for apothecary course and three of them passed in 1852. In 1860 Prof. Harkishan Singh was appointed as compounder in Calcutta Medical College. At around 1874 Madras Medical College started chemist and druggist course and in 1898 this medical college organize a separate department of druggist and chemist. In around 1939 Madras Medical College started two years B.Sc course in Pharmacy. In the same era in 1932 Prof. M. L. Schroff started pharmacy education in Banaras Hindu University conducting course B.Sc. Pharmacy. Prof. M. L. Schroff is called as pioneer of pharmacy education in India. Prior to 1932 the need of hospital pharmacist was fulfilled by training the pharmacist in medical stores which were known as compounders. In 1937 Government of Madras sanctioned a post of Pharmacist at Government General Hospital, Madras who is involved in training of the compounder and takes care of dispensary. In 1941 Mr. S. H. Merchant was appointed as a hospital pharmacist in K. E. M. Hospital, Bombay and he is considered as first qualified graduate hospital pharmacist. The trend of appointing hospital pharmacist was established by K. E. M. hospital and was followed by other leading hospitals at that time like Maulana Azad Medical College New Delhi, The Jaslok Hospital Mumbai, Sir J. J. Hospital and Nair Hospital Mumbai etc.

Till 1960 the services in hospital pharmacy were pathetic and unacceptable. The compounders were working as hospital pharmacist. Many hospitals were of good standard but the hospital pharmacy services were very poor. The pharmacists were using mortar and pestle for compounding the medicaments. The preparations were dispensed in the bottles brought by patients themselves. They were not labeled and patients were invented to recognize their own bottles. After that the significant development in hospital pharmacy took place but is limited to the government, missionary hospital or other charitable hospitals in India. In 1966 Dr. Carl Flesch from Hungary, Switzerland served in India as a chief pharmacist in CMC Hospital Ludhiana and he was their till 1969.

The Pharmacy act was established in 1948 for overall development and control of pharmacy education and training and development of pharmacy practice in India. The Pharmacy Council of India was constituted as per the provision of Pharmacy Act 1948 and is now regulating and controlling the pharmacy education, training and registration of pharmacist in India. Later in 1960 to 1970 a large number of hospitals established a modern hospital pharmacy departments and services and appointed qualified hospital pharmacist in it. Today large number of post graduates and doctoral degree holders are working as hospital pharmacists in Indian Hospitals. The D. Pharmacy, B. Pharmacy and M. Pharmacy are the approved courses by Pharmacy Council of India to become a registered pharmacist, Diploma in Pharmacy is minimum qualification in India. The M. Pharmacy (post graduate course) has many specializations like Pharmaceutics, Quality assurance, Pharmaceutical Chemistry, Pharmaceutical Analysis, Clinical Pharmacy, Pharmacology, Pharmacy Practice and Pharmacognosy etc. Recently in 2008, Pharm. D (a six year integrated course) is also introduced by Pharmacy Council of India, New Delhi as a qualification for registered pharmacist. Maharashtra is the first state in India to introduce the Pharm. D course in Government institute at Government College of Pharmacy, Aurangabad and Amravati. Today in India there are more than 6 lakhs of registered pharmacists working as professionals. There were 6 registered pharmacists per 10000 populations. The pharmacist: population ratio is around 1: 1840 and around 1 pharmacist per physician.

As per The Pharmacy Act 1948, Pharmacy Council of India controls the qualification to become a registered pharmacist, minimum qualification required for admission to the courses to become a registered pharmacist, period and other details of practical training to be taken, syllabus of qualification, various conditions to be fulfilled by the institute for approval to run a course necessary for registration of pharmacist (D. Pharm., B. Pharm. or Pharm. D.) as per section 12. It also prescribes conditions to be fulfilled by the examination authority for conducting of examinations and conditions to be fulfilled by the practical training centre. The central council related to The Pharmacy council of India includes following members as per section 3

- Teachers
- Central Government
- Medical Council of India
- Director General, Health Services, ex-officio
- Drug Controller of India, ex-officio
- Director of Central Drug Laboratory, ex-officio
- University Grant Commission and AICTE, New Delhi
- State Pharmacy Council
- State Government

Hospitals

Illness constrains the human individual to restrict his activities and modify his way of life. Clinic is the place, area or facility where individual or group of physicians see the ambulatory patients for diagnosis and treatment by appointment. It is the site where patients are not admitted and almost all the patients are outpatients. The facility established by hospital for outpatient department is also known as clinic. The hospital is the facility where the patients can be admitted for the short term or long term treatment. The outpatients are also seen and treatment is given.

The purpose of establishment of hospitals in ancient days was religious rather than medical care. The socially isolated, mentally retarded, age old, physically handicapped, socially depressed, sick, weak and neglected individuals were sent in these hospitals and kept outside of society. The individuals were isolated from their relatives and friends and send in these exclusive places meant for that purpose only.

During the episodes of epidemic communicable diseases, camps were used to house the patients away from society so that communicable diseases (like tuberculosis, cholera, leprosy etc.) should not spread. In later era a separate special facilities were created for admission of such patients away from society known as hospitals which were the first origin of hospitals.

In India hospitals were established after introduction of modern system of medicine, till that the Indian hospitals were ashrams. In 18th century hospitals were harsh and unhygienic. The area where patients were kept was dirty. No anesthetics or antibiotics were used during surgery. Nursing care was done by weak, age old, incompetent persons. Before the Independence the total numbers of hospitals in India were around 7500 with bed occupancy around one lakh. In post-independence era the health care facility, infrastructure and man power was developed.

The Bhore committee in 1946 introduced the concept of primary health care as a basic unit close to the people for integrated curative and preventive health care to the rural population. The health planner in India has visualized PHC and its sub center as a proper infrastructure to provide health services to the rural population. The central council of health in its first meeting on January 1953 recommended the establishment of PHCs. Bureau of Indian Standards (BIS) has prescribed standards for hospitals. Under the National Rural Health Mission (NRHM), Indian Public Health Standards has framed Community Health Centre. For providing optimal quality health care a standard has been recommended for PHC called as "Indian Public Health Standards (IPHS) for PHCs". The objectives of IPHS are to provide comprehensive primary health care to community through PHCs, to achieve and maintain acceptable standards of quality care and to make the service more responsive to the need of the community. The overall objective of IPHS is to provide health care that is quality oriented and sensitive to the needs of community.

As per IPHS the minimal assured services required in PHCs includes medical care, maternal and child health care, family planning, medical termination of pregnancy, management of reproductive tract infections, nutrition services, school health, adolescent health care, promotion of safe drinking water and basic sanitation, prevention and control of local endemic diseases like malaria, cholera, dysentery etc., disease surveillance and control, collection and reporting of vital events, education about health, national health program, referral services, training, basic laboratory services, monitoring and supervision, AYUSH services, rehabilitation, 24 hr delivery services and new born care, selected surgical procedures, recording of vital events etc.

The modern hospitals are institutes for care, cure, treatment, diagnosis, rehabilitation of sick, injured individuals and these centers are also used for studying diseases and training the doctors, nurses, clinical and hospital pharmacists. A personal care of patient is taken. Hospitals have gain a professional attitude providing best services in health care. These hospital aims at speedy recovery of patients with minimal cost and best facility. The ancillary luxurious facilities like air conditioner, telephone, newspaper etc. are provided at bed site.

These hospitals depending upon various factors can be classified in various categories. They can be classified on the basis of ownership and management they run. These classifications include Government hospital, Military hospital, Private hospital, Cooperative hospital and Charitable hospital. Depending on the pathway practice they follow in the hospital for treating patients can be classified as Allopathic hospital, Ayurvedic hospital, Siddha, Unani hospitals etc. Based on specialization they can be classified as multi-specialty, cardiology, cancer and eye hospital etc. The hospitals can also be classified on the basis of size and bed capacity. Depending on the purpose, the hospitals can be categorized as teaching hospitals, rehabilitation centers etc. and on the basis of level of health care facilities provided they can be primary, secondary or tertiary health care centers. After considering all these contributing factors, hospitals can be classified as (following different types as) follows:

- **Government hospital:** The expenses incurred for the construction, building, development, management and maintenance of the hospital were borne by the government of the concerned state or central govt. the salary of medical professionals and other health care persons like nursing staff, pharmacist are paid by government. The cost of treatment of the patients is borne by government or it is provided at vary minimal cost which meets the operational cost of the instruments and facilities. Government also established large hospital in collaboration with private agencies on public private partnership (PPP) basis. The objective of establishment of these hospitals is also to provide good health care facility with minimal cost.

- **Health care centre:** The health care centers are also governed and run by government for providing health care facilities at rural population level. Primary health care center has a general practitioner, a nurse and a hospital pharmacist at the local center and provide health care facilities. These hospitals are based at village level. The secondary health care center provides the health care of specialist in terms of hospital facility and physician. The patients referred by primary health care centers or directly accessed patients are treated at secondary health care centers. These hospitals are based at taluka place. The tertiary or higher health care centers are more complex and have sophisticated facility with more flit of specialists. The physician of secondary health care center refers the patients to this hospital. These hospital work on regional basis like district hospital, civil hospital etc. The facilities like catheterization laboratory, open heart surgery, transplantation, orthopedic are available in these hospitals.
- **Military hospitals:** The military hospitals were established to take care of the casualties arises in military operations. The trend of military hospital was started way back during world wars. The Indian Army Medical Corps (IAMC) was formed during World War II. The IAMC was formed as a merger of various other medical organizations like Indian Medical Services (IMS), The Indian Medical Department (IMD) and The Indian Hospital Corps (IHC). The idea of organizing medical services and formation of IAMC came in to existence during outbreak of World War II. The administrative head quarter of IAMC was at Pune in 1943. The Armed Force Medical Services were established in 1949 as head service for Army, Navy and Air Force. In 1950 IAMC was re-designated as Army Medical Corps. In 1962 The Armed Force Medical College (AFMC) came in to existence, it is a premier medical institute and training center for undergraduate and post graduate medical students. Now-a-days it is well known as AFMC catering the need of military and civil health care as on today.
- **General hospitals:** General hospitals were established to take care of the wide and common issues of the health problems in the society. These hospitals provide services for diagnosis and

treatment. The critical cases and the medical patients which require special facility for the treatment are forwarded to the other hospitals by general hospital. General hospital provides an immediate first site treatment to the patients.

- **Teaching hospitals:** In India teaching hospitals are established as part of medical college. The Medical Council of India (MCI) governs and regulates the norms and standards for these types of hospitals and colleges. They are also known as medical college and hospital or hospital and training institute. These institute trains the students for diploma, degree and based on that the MCI or respective state council will grant license for the medical practice as per Indian Medical Council Act 1956. The specialized training is also given to the medical students in specialized treatment like surgery, dentistry, pediatrics etc. The establishment of such hospitals and training institutes/medical colleges is regulated by MCI Regulation 1999. Such hospitals also work as research center, where facilities are created for study of specific aspect of the disease, clinical trials etc., and various system of medicine is integrated for benefits of patients.
- **Special hospital:** Now days the health care practice is more of specialty rather than general medical practice. The old concept of therapy is popular as general medical practice (GMP), which is not practiced in modern era of specialty hospital where treatment of diseases are more focused rather than general. The GMP is cost effective but priority is given to the more focused and specialized treatment having highest sophisticated techniques for the treatment in specific diseases in special hospitals. The concept of special hospitals are popular on name of the disease, organ or system affected like eye hospital, cancer hospital, diabetes hospital, tuberculosis hospital, obstructive and gynecology hospital, orthopedic hospital, maternity hospital etc. The disadvantage of specialty hospital is that patients suffering from other than specific diseases have to be referred to other hospital. Orthopedic patient cannot be treated in maternity hospital or a cancer patient cannot be admitted in tuberculosis hospital. However, the special hospital has all the facilities required for treatment of specific diseases.
- **Multispecialty hospitals:** Multispecialty hospitals are similar to that of specialty hospital and have additional advantage that

in the same hospital more than one specialty facilities are available. It only involves referring the patient from one department to other rather than to the other hospital. The multispecialty hospital also has sophisticated facilities as that of specialty hospital but in multiple special areas of treatments. The common specialty available in multispecialty hospital includes neurology, cardiology, ENT, ophthalmology, pediatrics, orthopedics, dermatology, psychiatry etc.

- **Private hospitals:** A non-government organization is responsible for management, administration and ownership of the private hospital like some individual, private company, firm, cooperative society, charitable trust or religious organization. Private hospitals may be of profit oriented. In recent years private hospitals have contributed a lot in health care system. The cost of treatment in private hospital might be high as compared to other hospitals but better services can be obtained at affordable cost. A large number or chain of hospitals of specialty hospitals, multispecialty hospitals have been established by private sector. These hospitals are localized in big cities. Major Corporate of India like TATA group, Hinduja group, Reliance, Wockhardt, Escorts, Apollo are significantly involved in the setting up of hospitals. These hospitals are based in cities like Mumbai, New Delhi, Calcutta, Chennai etc. The Hospitals like Hinduja National Hospital and Medical Centre was established in 1953 and is amongst the best hospital in India till date. The Wockhardt group, Apollo group has started trend of chain hospitals in India.

  The hospitals like The Amrita Institute of Medical Science and Research Centre (AIMS) Kochi started in 1993 has a world class ultra-modern facility for cardio vascular diseases. The hospital like All India Institute of Medical Science, New Delhi (AIIMS) has a world class facility and name in the health care practice. Private hospital groups has also a tie-up with other groups which are not involved in health care business like ONGC, Indian Oil Corporation, Bharat Heavy Electricals etc.

- **Cooperative hospitals:** A group of persons having common interest come together to establish a social services and established a cooperative hospitals. These hospitals are nonprofit making institutes and organization provides health care facility at comparatively affordable cost. They play important role in providing low cost treatment for illness to the lower and middle strata of society. The cooperative hospitals were established from funds raised and collected through shares and shareholders. More health benefits are passed to the shareholders. The governments also encourage the establishment of cooperative hospitals by providing subsidy in building, taxes, subscriptions, loans etc. The ultimate goal of establishing such hospitals is to provide a low cost medical facility to the affordable class of society who cannot afford the cost of medical expenses.

- **Rehabilitation centers:** Rehabilitation centers are the institutes where facilities for treatment of chronic diseases available. It's more of care taking unit rather than a hospital. The facilities for diagnosis, treatment and services for specific conditions are provided to the patients. Hospitals for physically handicapped, alcoholism treatment, geriatric hospitals can be termed as a rehabilitation centers. The patients has to stay in hospital for prolong period of time for treatment.
- **System of practice hospitals:** This is a category of hospital where a particular system of medicinal therapy is followed. Modern hospitals practice the allopathic system of medicine for the treatment. Ayurvedic hospitals are hospitals where ayurvedic system of medicine is practiced. The Hospitals prescribing homeopathic medicines are known as homeopathic hospitals. Similarly other system of medicine like unani system, siddha system, physiotherapy, Chinese system, acupuncture system, aromatherapy are also practiced in various types of hospitals which are bases in particular system of practice.

Ward Round Participation

Ward round is a visit of medical practitioner alone or along with team member involved in health care professional at the bedside of the patient to review health status and follow-up. The health care professional team involves medical students, Pharm. D students, hospital pharmacist, nursing staff, junior staff etc. Usually one ward round is conducted every day to review the progress in health of patients. More than one round may also be conducted within day if needed, such multiple ward round depends on the health status of the patients. Critically ill patients in intensive care unit require continuous monitoring and junior medical practitioner may be deputed for continuous supervision of patients. Pharmacist's participation in ward round was initiated at around 1970 in United States and United Kingdom.

The participation of pharmacist in ward round will help in promoting the rational use of drug and decrease the adverse drug events. It will improve patients care and reduce length of stay and ultimately health care cost involved in treatment. The ultimate objective of hospital pharmacist in ward round participation is to understand the patients clinical status and progress towards currently planned and given therapy and therapeutic goals. This will provide relevant information on various aspects of therapy such as pharmacology, pharmacokinetics, bioavailability, pharmacodynamics of drug administered, drug availability and cost, drug interaction and adverse drug reactions etc. It also helps in detection, management and prevention of adverse drug reactions and drug interactions. Through ward round participation pharmacist also helps in in-patients discharge planning. It also help pharmacist to understand how drugs elucidates their effect and leading to improvement in patients condition.

Depending on the purpose and composition of health care professionals the ward round is classified as:

- Pre-round
- Registrar/Resident round
- Professor/chief round
- Teaching round

Pre-round is conducted by medical post graduate students in teaching hospitals. No or very few management decisions are taken during this round. The trainee clinical pharmacists usually join along with interns and post graduate students in this round. They study and complete the patient's medication, medication history and clinical review at this time. In teaching hospital, registrar and residential individuals also conduct the ward round along with other management representatives. This round is conducted at least once a day at fixed timing, usually in morning. Non-medical managerial decisions are taken during this round. Clinical pharmacist participate in this round to gain the managerial and management experience. In teaching hospital the chief medical officer or professor in specialty conduct the chief round also known as professor round. This round is for review of patients for their health condition and improvement in health status. The round is conducted for all the patients under care on daily basis and if needed (in critical patients) twice a day. This round is most challenging for pharmacist to gain the clinical knowledge and experience. Academic medical staff conducts the bedside clinical teaching during this round. This teaching is conducted for graduate, post graduate, residential medical students and interns of the hospital. This round is usually extensive and conducted few times weekly. This round provides opportunity to the pharmacist to improve the clinical knowledge.

Pharmacist need to prepare well before ward round participation. Accurate and up-to-date information should be kept regarding patient's history, health status, disease management, medication etc. for effective participation in the ward round. Review of medication chart, case record, should be completed before attending ward round. Participation of pharmacist in pre-ward round gives idea of overview of drug treatment and related issues that arise during ward round with professors. It gives pharmacist idea and priority fixing of drug related problem. It prepares pharmacist with remedial actions for identified drug related problems. It helps to maintain patients profile and summarize the information related to the patient's drugs therapy.

Pharmacist must complete pre-ward round well ahead of the commencement of professors and teaching round. Pharmacist should set a priority to those rounds he wants to contribute. Many large hospitals have large numbers of different round and it is not necessary that pharmacist should contribute in all ward rounds. If hospital has formulary for drug prescriptions and other guidelines, pharmacist should ensure that all the prescriptions are given according to hospital formulary. Pharmacist should carry appropriate references like BNF, CIMS, and Drug review, along with him while working in the ward round. Pharmacist should avoid entering in the discussion of physician regarding diagnosis. The pharmacist's intervention should directly result in change in patient's therapy. The intervention of pharmacist in assisting prescribing can be of several forms. Active involvement results from use of guidelines passive involvement by drug information services and reactive involvement by monitoring prescriptions.

The major intervention by pharmacist during ward round participation arise related to dose and frequency of administration, choice of medicament for treatment, adverse effects expected and reported, drug interactions, formulation preferred for administration, duration of drug therapy, action, use and pharmacology of active medicament, availability and supply of drug for treatment, patients medication, legal and administrative issues raised, other issues such as storage of drugs etc.

Good professional relations, effective communication skills, thorough clinical knowledge of drugs are the pre-requisites of effective ward round participation by pharmacist. Pharmacist must try to resolve difference of opinion if any directly but in respectful manner. Knowledge of local/regional language will help in communicating between health care professional and help pharmacist to interacting effectively with patients. Pharmacist should take caution while discussing issues related to patients during ward round and strictly avoid bluffing or guessing and must retrieve the information and then communicate it to the concerned. Pharmacist should not challenge the integrity of the health care professionals.

Pharmacists come across various issues during ward round which requires follow up. These issues includes

- **Enquiries:** Unanswered queries raised by any professional during ward round must be recorded and a follow up of it must be communicated as early as possible. The solution may be communicated by any mode like telephone, fax, e-mail, written document, printout or in person.
- **Information:** Appropriate information needed by medical health professionals must be communicated in time, regarding issues raised by them like change in therapy etc.
- **Documentation:** Any recommendations, suggestions, intervention and changes thereafter made by physician must be documented appropriately in appropriate language. This documentation must be appropriately done during ward round or immediately after the ward round.
- **Alteration in plan:** Pharmacist may feel need to alter the plan of patients care to meet the need of patients management.

Pharmacist must discuss with patients regarding process of treatment if needed.

Drug and Poison Information Services

Providing the drug information is fundamental responsibility of Pharmacist irrespective of other commitment as a pharmacist. Drug information and poison information services are the specialized services present and provided in hospital or at any other place where the unbiased, well referenced and critically evaluated information on any aspect of drug or poison is provided. The centers that render these services are known as drug information center (DIC) and poison information center (PIC) or Poison control centers (PCC). The drug and poison information services have a system for organizing; dissemination of drug information as and when required to person who needs it. The components of information provided by drug information services comprises of dose, schedule, therapeutic effects, pharmacokinetics, adverse drug reaction, allergic reactions, drug and food interactions, availability and substitute, administration in pregnancy and lactation, poisoning and toxicity of drugs etc. The DIC gives information regarding Right drug in Right dose or Right dosage form by Right route to the Right patient. The poison information service provides information about poisoning management, immediate information on early diagnosis, treatment, management, of poisoning. PIC is a specialized area of DIC which provides information regarding, animal toxins and even therapeutic drugs. It also provides information regarding other toxic agents like plants, mushrooms, insects, snakes, spiders and stings.

Drug Information Centers (DIC)

The term DIC evolves at around 1960 and in 1962 first pharmacist operated DIC was established at Kentucky, USA. In 1964 first conference on drug information services was held and in 1969. A specialized DIC was established at London Hospital UK and Leeds general Infirmary. In 1975 The Mills Commission Report describes the main function of pharmacist as drug information provider. DIC in India is still in infancy stage. There are around 15 DIC all over India. Karnataka State Pharmacy Council, Trivandrum Medical College and Ramakrishna Hospital are amongst those who established DIC first in India. The established DIC may be of three types depending on the organization they operated and governed by 1. Hospital based DIC, 2. Industry based DIC and 3. Community based DIC.

The need of DIC intensifies because of new drug and new treatment models being introduced, explosion of biomedical information, multiplicity and complexity of drug. Many therapeutic guidelines have been published by various organization and selection of appropriate regimen for treatment become critical. The complex nature of drug information and its interaction with other drug, food material and herbal medicine make it more complex. The health care professionals have become more educated and professional regarding therapeutic agents. They expect that the therapeutic regimen must be safe as possible. But the day to day introduction of new drugs and updating the information of older drugs lack the adequacy of information. Limited availability of current literature, inappropriateness of documentation also contributes in it. The rational selection and utilization of drug becomes a problem, updating the information to health care professional is need of time. A large number of clinical trials going on new drugs also added more information in this. Pharmaceutical industry may provide biased information for promotion of their product. In such condition only the DIC can provide appropriate information to the health care professionals which will be unbiased in relation to all of the above facts. To do this, pharmacist can provide link between information and health care professionals through DIC.

Drug information center provides current information which will be critically evaluated in particular type of patient and situation of treatment. DIC provides specialized facility for information providing to those who need it in unbiased manner and in systematic approach. The information provided is unbiased, critically evaluated and up-to-date, patients specific, with integration of new technology, and have the ability to change the environment of health care system. The organization of DIC will depends on type of activity done and offers as services, space available for establishing such services, budget, staff and resources. As per the policy decisions DIC may also provide services like answering in-house calls of the hospital health care professional, assisting in establishing and updating the hospital formulary, participation in drug use evaluation programs, coordination in adverse drug reaction monitoring and reporting services, coordination and contribution in newsletters, may work or assist in pharmacy and therapeutic committee, etc.

Sources of information: Providing the unbiased and accurate information through DIC will help physician in many ways. But this help depends on the source of information where from it was obtained. The source of information in DIC is categorized in three different types depending on source of information.

- **Primary source:** Primary source of information is most authentic and accurate source of information. Journal containing original articles in reputed journals with citation index and impact factor are primary source of information. Clinical trials and research articles from medical and pharmaceutical journals will be obtained. These articles are most updated and best source of information. This source is time consuming and costly.
- **Secondary source:** For the secondary source indexing and abstracting services like IDIS, IOWA, PUBMED, EMBASE, MEDLINE and Drug Information Services are the source of information. This source is quite useful and used for selective screening of primary literature. This source is also quite expensive for procurement and difficult to maintain. The source is limited to abstract only and no details are available.
- **Tertiary source:** For the information DIC also depends on tertiary source which includes standard text books and references. This includes AHFS Drug Information (American Society of Health-System Pharmacists USA), Martindale, The Complete Drug Reference, Indian Pharmacopoeia (I.P.), U.S.P., B.P., B.N.F., Computer database like micromedex etc. The information is available in composite, condensed and compact form. The information is easy and convenient to access and is mostly used source of information. But this information is little age old and lags behind than journals and abstract. Several years passes to publish these books and references.
- **Alternate source:** Internet, electronic bulletin boards, bulletins and other publications are the alternate source for DIC. Internet provides the ability to search the information recently published and discussed in media. This is not a reliable source of information and contains unregulated and biased health care information. The authenticity of site, peer reviewed retrieval; evaluation of facts must be done critically before taking the information in to account. Electronic Bulletin

Board like ClinNet, PharmLine, PharmNet helps in monitoring drug related issues. Peer reviewed articles is not an authentic and reliable source of information. Bulletins, formularies, treatment guidelines, government and regulatory authority publications are also the source of alternate information.

Systemic Approaches to provide Drug Information

While giving the information through DIC pharmacist should never guess the information, ethical issues related to the information must be considered like patients privacy, misuse of patients or physicians information etc. Before delivering, the information must be organized. The information must be tailor made and should be provided as per need and nature of patient disease. Pharmacist must disclose the source of information where from obtained. The information provided should be comprehensive and there should not be any delay in providing information. Even if there is any delay it must be informed. During answering the queries from DIC a stepwise approach must be used. This will help in understanding the pharmacist exact nature of information needed; it will reduce the literature survey time and also avoid overlooking significant information. The basic steps are involved in answering drug information queries includes:

- **Detail information about requester:** Details of information regarding the requester must be obtained before proceeding to gather the information. The details of information regarding regular requester must be available with the database and pharmacist should not spend time in gathering this information. From the requester pharmacist must guess the depth and nature of information required. An experienced and senior physician requires concise and to the point information while trainee and junior physician will require every details of the information. Deadline for the information required must be obtained to see the emergency of information to be provided. Pharmacist has to manage timing in providing such information time to time. For the new requester the details of information like name, address, location, position, and mode by which information can be delivered must be asked. This information must be stored and used for further requests from same requester.

- **Background information procurement:** An experienced pharmacist by his/her communication and asking question skillfully procures necessary background information for searching the information. This is in aim of determining ultimate question to be answered by him. This questioning is most critical to prepare a good search strategy and to find out exact key word for searching. The background information is needed for assessing that whether the request is concerned to specific patient or academic in nature. This will help in developing search strategy and narrowing the search of more precise information.
- **Category of information needed:** After obtaining the request, it must be understood and categorized before starting search strategy. All the aspects must be understood before seeking answer. The information regarding medical terminology, pathological data, disease condition etc. must be assessed and evaluated. This exercise will reduce the estimated time and achieve more acceptable information. This is important because the entire search must be focused to answer the queries of the requester.
- **Determining search strategy:** After finalizing the need of requester take into account the available information resources and priorities them on the basis of emergency, severity, location and requester of information. The search must begin with tertiary source and then progress to secondary and primary source of information. The searching must be stopped when desired information is obtained. Record the resource and summarize the information before forwarding to the requester.
- **Obtaining and interpreting data:** The information thus obtained must be evaluated critically for consistency between various sources. Whether the clinical observation is relevant to large population or found in specific patient only. Absolute answers to the queries received are rare and hence whenever possible details of full text must be provided with the information. There might be lack of data or conflict in the information searched. This must be summarized during answering the queries.

- **Composing and providing information:** Establish outline for the information obtained in response to the request received. The answer must be composed after critical evaluation of data obtained in search. The answer must be provided with rapid and point wise concise information at the end of document. Busy clinician prefers to read the concise information but the detailed information must be provided if required by the clinician. During written communication answer to the request must be raised first with detailed information and concise ending of the document. If request is to be replied with telephonic call then main point must be stated and marked before making an answer call. For detail call detailing and record keeping can be done at later stage and answer must be communicated first.
- **Follow-up and documentation:** Follow-up of information provided gives appropriateness of information. If the DIC is in the same hospital where the information is forwarded then follow-up becomes easy. The outcomes of the information provided must be determined. These outcomes and feedbacks must be recorded in log book, computer document or any other mode. Busy practitioner of DIC may lack in follow-up, documentation and will lose a valuable information regarding advice provided by him to the medical practitioners.
- **Quality assurance of data provided:** Establishing a quality assurance mechanism in DIC is difficult task. The flow of information is from lower authorities to the higher authorities. There is no reason higher authority is answerable to lower authority for providing feedback system or quality assurance mechanism. Still quality assurance program is an integral part of DIC and will provide additional information and knowledge to the DIC pharmacist's opportunity to learn, update the knowledge and provide guideline for future development. The quality assurance can be evaluated in terms of resources available in DIC and standard operating procedures following during answering queries.

Poison Information Centers (PIC)

PIC is also termed as Poison Control Center (PCC). During World War II large number of chemicals and drug molecules were introduced and as a consequence there were high incidences of poisoning. In European countries at late 1940 special wards were established for treatment of poisoning cases. At around 1949 PIC was started in Netherland and UK. In India PIC are essential as poisoning is major cause of death. As per WHO report in year 2000 unintentional poisoning is ninth major cause of death globally and sixth most common cause in India in young adults. At around 2010 there were only four WHO recognized PIC in India. The first National Poison Information Centre was established in 1994 at All-India Institute of Medical Science (AIIMS), New Delhi. Other centers were located at National Institute of Occupational Health Ahmadabad, Government General Hospital Chennai, Amrita Institute of Medical Science and Research Cochin. Looking to the scenario of poisoning cases this much PIC centers is not at all able to meet the demand of poisoning information in India.

PIC is a specialized area of DIC that provides information regarding toxic effects of various chemicals and medicine including toxins from plant, insects and other sources. PIC provides information regarding diagnosis, management, treatment, prevention and hazard management of poisoning with any substance. It's binding to the PIC to timely provide information regarding poisoning and its management. PIC service deals with risk assessment, diagnosis management and prevention of exposure of poison. The main aim of PIC is to prevent mortality, morbidity, improve quality related to health, reduce cost of treatment of poisoning and also reduces hospitalization period. There is absolute necessity that the information provided by PIC should have immediate access in order to achieve function effectively. The information is given most of the time telephonically and instantaneously within few minutes. For PIC professional to provide this vital information accurately, timely, must have all component of this service and competency to handle these cases.

The role of PIC can be denoted as providing poison information services, management of poisoning cases, analytical services for toxicological substances, toxico-vigilance, conducting training, education and awareness programs for healthcare professionals, development of treatment protocol for poison management. The PIC provides following information.

- Toxicological information about drugs, chemicals and other material
- Adverse drug reaction information
- Information regarding drug-drug and drug-food, interactions
- Bioavailability information of drugs and products
- Compatibility information
- Drug induce disease information
- Information regarding new drugs introduced
- Information regarding current trends in drug therapy
- Assist the hospital for selection of drugs for formulary
- Drug research literature evaluation
- Training of health care professionals and fellow pharmacists

Similar to that of DIC, PIC also get information from various sources which can be categorized as primary, secondary and tertiary. It is essential that PIC should have all types of sources available. PIC specialist should search and evaluate the information for its accuracy and consistency. Specialist should use all the skill for extracting accurate information from available resources in minimum possible time. The primary source of information includes journals of medicine or toxicity, toxicology, clinical toxicology, environmental toxicology etc., of high reputation and impact factor. The secondary source comprises of sources such as poison index, hypertox, toxbase, intox, toxinz etc. The tertiary information source includes standard text books of medicine, chemistry, pharmacology, animal and plant toxins etc., it also includes other books like Pharmacopoeia, National Formulary, list of agricultural and chemical products. The steps involved in receiving the query, obtaining the information and delivering the information is similar to that of DIC.

DIC *vs* PIC

Both DIC and PIC has common goal to provide the information in a comprehensive manner, accurate and timely to enhance the medical care of patient. A basic difference between DIC and PIC is the beneficiary for whom the information is collected and delivered. The DIC information is collected for the patients who need rapid recovery from disease. As compared to it PIC information is for person undergone unintentional or intentional poisoning. The need of information in DIC is time bound but need of information in PIC is urgent and must be delivered as quickly as possible. The end user for DIC may not be serious but the end user of PIC might be even struggling for life. DIC information is a specialized facility required for timely delivery of information whereas PIC should provide the information round the clock. In DIC the number and volume of call is less and specifically from health care professionals, whereas in PIC the large number of calls are generally from extremely large publics. The working pattern of DIC can be as normal office having duty hours and weekly holidays but PIC must work round the clock and round the year. The working and establishment cost of PIC is very high as compared to DIC. The number of staff required and their qualification for PIC is also much higher as compared to DIC. DICs are funded by hospitals, college or medical centers. On other hand PICs are funded by public/private organization, donation programs and industries.

Paediatric and Geriatric Pharmacy Practice

Anatomy and physiology of paediatric and geriatric patients are different from normal adult individuals. Organ functions, hemodynamic parameters, homeostasis, metabolic activity, functioning of excretory organs and system, physiological parameters are also quite different in paediatric and geriatric individuals. These differences make them different in their therapeutics also during drug therapy. A special wards and specialization in studies exist for pediatric patients but no such trends of special wards and specialization in medical exist for geriatric patients. This difference in anatomical and physiological status is vulnerable for drug therapy. The therapeutic regimens, alteration applicable for normal adult individuals may not be same for paediatric and geriatric patients.

The normal hematocrit in pediatric is much higher as compared to adult individual. The normal hematocrit ranges from 38 to 46% in adult female and 40 to 54% in adult male. In paediatrics the normal hematocrit is around 60 to 65%. This much hematocrit if observed in adult will be declared as patient of polycythemia, however the paediatrics with this hematocrit is considered as normal. The comparative calculated dose required for anesthetics and alcohols in therapy is significantly higher in paediatric patients than normal adult individuals because the metabolic status required for these drugs is quite high in pediatric patients, while geriatric patients requires comparative low dose when compared with normal adult individual because the metabolic status in geriatric patients is quite week when compared to adults. However the susceptibility of both paediatric and geriatric individuals for diseases and unexpected toxicity is high when compared to adults.

Paediatric Pharmacy Practice

As per survey in 2007 amongst the total world population 33% in paediatric populations. This population has a significant different anatomical, physiological and pathological status. The organs and functions are poorly developed and special care is required to be taken during their disease status. The death of children due to sulfanilamide elixir and birth defect in newborns due to thalidomide made us compulsory to look the paediatric patients in different way and establish special wards and faculty of medicine in the study.

Children are unique and different from adults in many ways. The requirement of dose of drug differs significantly per kilogram of body weight. The pharmacokinetic and pharmacodynamics parameters and status is also quite different. The comparative dose calculated from adult dose required per kilogram per day is higher in children and lower in infants. The type of dosage form required for pediatric patient is also different. Children are not comfortable with tablet or capsule dosage form and they required syrups or suspension which will be easier for them to swallow. Moreover children are afraid of injectables and may not cooperate during admission of such dosage forms.

Looking to all above factors the cost of paediatric pharmaceuticals is always higher than normal dosage form and different factors has to be considered during formulating paediatric dosage forms. Around 80% formulations of adults are different from paediatrics although they contains same medicament and used for same therapeutic purpose. A pharmacist in hospital pharmacy must consider all these factors during dealing with paediatric patients. They should complete a special training or additional course before practicing paediatric pharmacy. Additional skills and practice for management, clinical handling, should be acquired by pharmacist in paediatric pharmacy practice.

It should be understood that the children are small adults; they are not a mini adults. The scaled down dose of child from adult may not be appropriate or sufficient for paediatric patients. Many changes in body takes place when child grow to a adolescence like change in amount of water, protein, fat and muscular content. Changes also takes place in hormonal and enzymatic status of body leading to change in metabolic and dispositional status. These changes make the requirement of drug and its dose variable.

Factors like gender, heredity, diseases, prior exposure to drug therapy may also alter the pharmacokinetic and pharmacodynamics of paediatric patients. Knowledge of pharmacokinetics and pharmacodynamics must be acquired by the hospital pharmacist to handle paediatric patients. Pharmacist have to play vital role in immunization programs like pulse polio. Pharmacist can work also with health care professional team in identifying the patient educating and motivating them for immunization. They can determine the need and work as facilitator in immunization programs. Pharmacist can also work for monitoring after effect of immunization, efficacy, schedule and monitoring.

Geriatric Pharmacy Practice

A term elderly referred to peoples with age group more than 65 years. Geriatrics is the branch of science or medicine which deals with medication, social, health care and illness related issues of elder individuals. Changes in geriatric individuals occur gradually and differ from patient to patients. The age of 65 years and above used in definition of geriatrics is arbitrary. Sometime in this group individual aged 60 or above is also included. The improvement in health, hygiene, quality health care services, housing etc. has decreased the mortality rate in geriatrics as well as paediatric individuals. In developed countries during 1900 the population of geriatrics were only around 2%, which was increased to more than 13% by year 2000 and it is predicted that it will increased to 20% by the year 2050. In developing country increased in percent population of geriatric patients is slower. In India, during 2006 around 8% population was in geriatric category and by the year 2050 this percentage is expected to increase up to 21%. The contribution of pharmacist in rational use of drugs, safe and error free use of medications, effective monitoring of adverse drug reaction improved the quality and life span of geriatric individuals. Presently around 60 million geriatric peoples exist in India.

Very age old geriatric patients of more than 75 years old are more sensitive to the effect of drugs and this is due to physiological changes that occur due to advancement in the age resulting in change in pharmacokinetics and pharmacodynamics behaviors of drugs in their body. These changes make them more prone for adverse effects, adverse drug reactions and comparatively require small dose when compared to adult individuals. Prescribing the geriatric patients with normal dosage form leads to inappropriate prescribing. There should be reduced dose prescription for geriatric patients. Forgetfulness also contributes in complications associated with treatment of geriatric patients. Patient may forget that he/she has taken a drug and may repeat the dose leading to double administration or he/she may not at all take the drug leading to poor therapeutic action.

Aging leading to alteration in pharmacokinetics includes altered absorption, distribution, metabolism, elimination whereas change in pharmacodynamics includes change in drug receptor sensitivity, change in homeostasis etc. The renal clearance rate and glomerular filtration in geriatrics decreased up to 50%. The geriatric patients with renal failure require special attention and significant alterations in the treatment. There is significant decrease in renal elimination of drugs which are excreted through renal route. Decline hepatic function with age reduces the enzymatic system and metabolism. The rate of clearance by hepatic metabolism decreases. With progressed age rate at which drug is absorbed alters significantly. Rate of drug absorption is decreased significantly where as the extent to which drug is absorbed remains same. The first pass metabolism decreases due to reduced blood flow to liver. Reduction in total body water and body mass and increase in fat affects distribution of drug. Lipid soluble drugs are deposited in tissues and fat which increases distribution and prolongs duration of action.

Change in responsiveness to the drug is due to alteration in pharmacodynamic changes. There is alteration in receptor sensitivity, and receptor binding of drug. The significant loss of CNS cells leads to adverse effects to drugs like benzodiazepines. Loss of cholinergic neurons in selective pathway reduces memory and state of confusion. There is increased level of catecholamine metabolizing enzymes like MAO and reduces the biological amount of neurotransmitters like dopamine, adrenaline and noradrenaline. This decline level of catecholamine is responsible for reduction in therapeutic effect of drug acting *via* them like antipsychotics.

Immobility, falls, osteoarthritis, osteoporosis, fracture, confusion, delirium, dementia, anemia, urinary and fecal incontinences are the common problems associated with geriatric patients. Taking in to account the above facts the multiple prescriptions of drugs in geriatric patients should be strictly avoided. The dose of prescribed drug should be altered by taking into consideration all the age related factors which contributes in modification of therapeutic effect. Drug should be avoided when giving of such drugs is associated with risk rather than benefits. Pharmacist should promote rational and safe use of drugs in geriatric patients. Pharmacist should pay extra attention while adjusting the dose, should minimize multiple prescribing, should identify and prevent adverse drug reactions.

Pharmacist should communicate with geriatric patients with consideration of their age and respect them. Impaired hearing, vision and cognition can be barriers of communication and they should be taken in to account while communicating with geriatric patients. Pharmacist should use simple techniques of talking lauder, with hand actions, going closer to them while talking, writing the instruction on a piece of paper in bold handwriting and simple language will help geriatric patient a lot. Pharmacist should always demonstrate ethical conduct with elders. Pharmacist should learn himself, and teach geriatric patient the various assistive techniques like stick, wheel chair, trolley, walking device etc. give simple tips and tricks to avoid falls in home and surrounding, take medicine review, monitor compliance.

Laboratory Data

The laboratory data may be of biochemical or hematological type. The laboratory data provides us to understand the patient's health and physiological function. Interpretation of laboratory data with confidence requires skill. Many clinical investigations depend on specific or non-specific laboratory investigations. These investigations are routinely accessed by clinicians for diagnosis of patient's condition. These clinical finding are directly related to the drug therapy hence pharmacist also has (consent) concerned with these laboratory data and its management. The laboratory data and reports are always presented along with reference range. The ranges represent the minimal and maximal limit for the laboratory data. These range may vary and depends on age, physical condition, gender etc. these ranges may be misleading if not properly understood. The result that went outside this range represents the abnormal condition, disease state or improper functioning of the organ or system. However the results within the normal limit do not guarantee for normal condition and vice versa. Abnormal observation also does not guarantee the presence of disease or illness. The laboratory investigational result may appear as abnormal despite of normal condition and this is termed as false positive. The result of laboratory investigation if indicates normal despite of illness then it is termed as false negative. Such false positive or negative results obtained due to artifact effect like errors procedure and improper steps followed during investigations. The presence of reference standard during investigation gives idea about such false results and will avoid errors that occur in clinical investigation.

The clinical pharmacist or hospital pharmacist must be able to interpret the laboratory data because this data will assist the physician in taking decisions for drug therapy and drug therapy is completely dependent on the findings of clinical data. The laboratory data will also give whether the drug therapy will be appropriate for the patient or requires change. The laboratory data gives idea about appropriateness of the drug prescribed to the patients on particular illness. For example, NSAIDs are prescribed for many conditions like inflammation, gout etc. but the patient with renal failure may require to change the drug or adjust the dose of existing drug because NSAIDs are primarily excreted by renal route and renal failure largely alter their excretion. The pharmacist has to play active role and learn a skill to handle the laboratory data. Pharmacists should make themselves familiar for information needed by the patient and interpretation of laboratory data which play active role in patients' health care system.

Drugs and their metabolites are excreted through renal route. Kidney plays important role in excretion. Impaired or reduced renal function is the condition when the renal clearance through kidney is significantly reduces. Some category of drug itself impairs or reduces the kidney function. Many laboratory investigation and data obtained their after gives idea about renal function. These tests and investigations are termed as renal function tests. From such data it is possible to detect the kidney function, degree and nature of damage. The laboratory investigation for renal function includes estimation of serum creatinine, urea, urea nitrogen, glomerular filtration rate (GFR) etc.

Creatinine is metabolic product of proteins and muscles in body. It does not play any important or physiological role in human body. Through kidney it is excreted by tubular secretion process. Tubular secretion is unique for creatinine. Estimation of serum creatinine gives idea about tubular secretion process of kidney. Impaired tubular secretion can be investigated using detection of elevated serum creatinine level in serum. In geriatric patients the reduced muscle mass is responsible for reduced creatinine level and despite of significant renal impairment the serum creatinine level may observed within normal range. Elevated serum urea, urea nitrogen, electrolyte is common with increased serum creatinine level.

GFR is useful tool in determining many aspects of renal functions. GFR determines the renal clearance of drug and metabolites. Alteration in GFR leads to change in serum concentration of drug. Modified GFR may also require altering the dose of drug. Elevated GFR increases clearance of drug at early rate and dose of drug to be administered should be increased accordingly. The decline GFR means decreased in clearance rate of kidney and reduction of dose is essential. The patients with such modified GFR require modification in dose. In geriatric patients the GFR is significantly low while in paediatrics the GFR is quite high. The corresponding calculation of dosage for paediatric or geriatric patients depending on body mass or age may be errors if renal function and GFR is not taken in to account during dose adjustment.

Laboratory investigation of the hepatic function is known as liver function tests (LFT). LFT is indicator of functional capacity of liver. Increased LFT is the indicator of hepatic damage more specifically hepatocytes. The parameters of LFT include various enzymes of liver that includes gamma glutaryltransferase, alkaline phosphatase, lactate dehydrogenase, bilirubin, alanine and aspartate aminotransferase etc. Presence of one of the enzyme in serum at elevated quantity indicates the damage to hepatocytes and release of cell enzymes in circulation. Elevated serum bilirubin indicates impaired take up of bilirubin in gall bladder from hepatic ducts. Elevation of one or more of the above mentioned enzymes is an indication of different conditions of liver like gallstone, hepatitis, cirrhosis, viral infections like hepatitis A, B or C, etc. For the hospital pharmacist monitoring of LFT is the way to detect the adverse effect of drug like drug induced hepatitis. This information pharmacist can use for dose adjustment of drug which induces or prone to induce the hepatitis. The drugs which are primarily metabolized and excreted through liver must be given with caution in the patients with impaired liver function. Blood glucose level is important parameter in the diagnosis, treatment, progress of disease and monitoring of diabetes mellitus. The long term hyperglycemia in the diabetic patients leads to serious complication like retinopathy, nephropathy etc. Long term control of diabetes is monitored using measurement of glycosylated hemoglobin (HbA_{1c}). Measurements of serum glucose level, urinary glucose level are the indicators of hyperglycemic condition of diabetic patient. With drug treatment also it is not possible to maintain the blood glucose level in normal range. However patients can significantly reduce the long term complications by avoiding sustain hyperglycemic condition. Pharmacists play an important role by patients counseling and patient's education for management of normal glucose level. He can educate and train the diabetic patients or relatives for appropriate use of glucometers for effective monitoring of blood glucose level and prevention of hyperglycemia. Pharmacist can also help and guide the diabetic patients in managing the blood glucose level using modified diet, exercise etc. The management of diabetic complications like diabetic foot, wound healing can be assisted by the pharmacist.

The estimation of hematological profile includes hemoglobin (Hb), red blood cell count (RBC), white blood cell count (WBC) and platelet count. Estimation of Hb and RBC is indicator for oxygen carrying capacity (OCC) of blood. Reduced Hb and RBC reduce OCC and condition is called as anemia. Depending on occurrence, source, and after effect anemia are of different types. Hb and RBC is the tool to estimate and differentiate anemia. WBC is the tool to estimate the leucocytes present in the blood. Leucocytes are of different types and plays different role in body. Elevated and decrease level of each type of leucocytes is indicator of different abnormal states like leucopenia, leukocytosis, neutrophilia, eosinophilia, monocytosis etc. These abnormal statuses are indicators of different diseases like bacterial infection, urinary infection, tuberculosis, meningitis, allergic reaction, parasitic infections etc. Slight elevation of platelet count is the indicator of condition like inflammatory reaction. Drugs like heparin, thiazide induces thrombocytopenia as a toxic reaction. The pharmacist through his skill can counsel the patients for various hematological abnormalities. Proper diet program can avoid and help in reducing anemic condition. Monitoring of WBC count by pharmacist will help clinician as a guide in response to the treatment of illness. Decrease WBC indicates improvement in the clinical condition. Drug induced thrombocytopenia can be avoided by replacing the drug. Pharmacist can assist physician in such alteration of drug therapy. The other hematological estimation includes erythrocyte sedimentation rate, C-reactive proteins, blood group estimation are useful in various health conditions.

Therapeutic Drug Monitoring

Therapeutic efficacy of drug depends on the availability of drug and its active metabolite in a specific quantity at the site of action or receptor site. This quantity available at the site of action is termed as bioavailability. The various pharmacokinetic and pharmacodynamic and pharmaceutical parameters influence bioavailability of drug. The knowledge of pharmacokinetic behaviors of drug molecule will help in optimizing the bioavailability and ultimately the therapeutic effect of drug. Along with therapeutic effect of drug molecule the patient will also get side effect of that drug molecules which are undesirable. A perfect balancing of dose is required to elucidate the desired therapeutic effect and avoid the side effect of drug molecules. The dose adjustment may be critical when the therapeutic index of drug is narrow. Trimming of the dosage regimen becomes essential by taking into consideration the individual patient.

Therapeutic drug monitoring (TDM) is valid tool for determining the serum concentration of drug and its active metabolite for optimizing the pharmacotherapy in order to reach balance between therapeutic effect occurred and occurrence of adverse effect. TDM enables the clinician for individualization of dosage regimen. All the patients differ significantly for their pharmacokinetics and pharmacodynamics effects. The therapeutic efficacy for the drug may vary due to this differentiation and requires modification in dose in order to get the optimum therapeutic benefit from drug molecule administered. Lack of control on concentration of drug molecule in body and its bioavailability prevents the patient's therapeutic response consistency. The variation in pharmacokinetics and pharmacodynamics are responsible for this variable clinical responsiveness. The pharmacokinetic and pharmacodynamic factors of patients cannot be controlled by clinician but the dosage regimen and pharmaceutical factors can be controlled for better therapeutic efficacy. TDM is used to estimate blood level of drug so that most effective dose can be determined with toxicity avoidance.

In early 1960s measurement of concentration of drug molecules in biological fluids like serum, tissue fluid, saliva etc. in very minute quantity like micrograms or nanograms was difficult. This is due to lack of specific and accurate measurement techniques. Development of sophisticated analytical techniques like HPLC, LC-MS, LC-MS/MS, GC, GC-MS, HPTLC, RIA, EIA have made it possible to analyze very minute quantity of drug molecule in the biological fluids. Advancement in chromatographic techniques leads to separation of drug molecules and their active metabolite from biological materials for their effective analysis. The hybrid techniques like LCMS provide chromatographic separation along with molecular detection of drug quantitatively as well as qualitatively. The unknown metabolite of drug molecule, their separation from parent drug molecule and biological fluid and its structural elucidation is now possible simultaneously using these sophisticated and advances analytical techniques.

TDM is blend of knowledge of therapeutics, pharmacology, adverse effects, pharmacokinetics, pharmacodynamics, laboratory techniques and clinical techniques side of drug molecule. TDM is measurement of serum concentration of drug molecule and its active metabolite responsible for therapeutic benefit of the patients. TDM involves three objectives 1. To attend desire pharmacological effect 2. To reach maximal effect in shortest possible time and 3. To decrease risk factors. TDM is requested for the following clinical considerations.

- TDM is essential for promoting the optimum drug treatment by maintaining drug and its active metabolite serum concentration within therapeutic range.

- TDM is applicable to those drugs which have direct relationship with drug concentration and therapeutic response.
- TDM is essential when therapeutic index of the drug is very low (e.g., digoxin). The margin between maximum effective concentration and minimum toxic level is narrow. Slight variation in therapeutic drug level may cross the toxic boundary and patient may land in danger zone.
- The drug may have variable therapeutic efficacy and variation depends on the patient's anatomical and physiological condition. Paediatric, adult and geriatric patient have significant difference in their anatomy, physiology as well as pathological status. Drug may show variable relationship in such variation and TDM become essential.
- Therapeutic dose of a drug is decided for large group of patients taking that drug. The significant variation of patients from this large representative group makes it essential to undergo TDM.
- Patients with altered pharmacokinetics due to disease like hepatic or renal insufficiency, burns and ICU patients requires TDM during treatment.
- TDM is possible and effective when there is no adequate clinical response to given dose of drug even if measurable serum concentration of drug is obtained from biological system.
- If patient complains about persistent side effect even at therapeutically normal dose, then TDM is essential.
- To minimize the risk of drug toxicity even though it is not observed TDM can be requested. Treatment of aminoglycoside requires TDM to avoid potential toxic effect like nephrotoxicity.
- Individualization of dose when dose response relationship is unpredictable due to pharmaceutical factors, then TDM is essential. Phenytoin follows non-linear kinetics. Increase dose increases serum concentration in uneven proportion.
- The problem related to unidentified medical complication leading to poor therapeutic efficacy can be resolved using TDM. To resolve the problem of patients with anti-epileptic drug therapy and showing episodes of epileptic attack, TDM is done.

- Other than pharmacotherapy TDM can also useful in identification, severity assessment of poisoning cases. The effective antidote treatment and rate of excretion will help the physician for better treatment of patients.
- The patients showing variable pharmacokinetic behaviors for drug absorption, distribution, metabolism and excretion produces poor correlation between dose response relationship and in such case to optimize the dose TDM become essential. The variable pharmacokinetics may be due to age, gender, pregnancy, lactation etc.
- In many condition the monitoring of clinical effect of drug on patient is difficult. The clinical effect is related to drug serum concentration. The efficacy of drug can only be assessed from TDM data. Prophylactic dosing of anticonvulsants, antidepressants drugs cannot be evaluated by their clinical effect.
- TDM become essential when therapeutically effective drug produces toxic metabolite.

For the effective and fruitful TDM process, it requires collaborative, multidisciplinary approach. Pharmacist has a vital role to play in TDM process. Pharmacist has a clinical skill along with traditional skill that can be used for rendering the TDM services. Pharmacist has knowledge of pharmacokinetic profile of drugs. Pharmacist is reliable and responsible person for giving information regarding the TDM services. Pharmacist can assist medical professionals in dose adjustment, dose calculations during TDM process. He can be a potential TDM team member amongst doctors, scientists, technical persons and nurses. Pharmacists can advise clinician in decision making of dose adjustment in patients who need such adjustment for their age, sex, disease condition etc. He can also assist clinician in appropriate use and timing of TDM and interpretation of TDM results. Pharmacist can also provide background information of patient like allergic condition, associated disorders, other pathological condition, comprehensive medical history etc. Pharmacist has significant knowledge about analytical measurement of drug using various sophisticated analytical tools. This skill, pharmacist can use during analysis and interpretation of TDM data obtained. In addition to this pharmacist may also involve in:

- Decision making about dose, dosing interval, dosage form, route of drug administration for individual patients in view of age, sex, body weight, race, metabolic status, renal and hepatic function of the patient.
- Adjusting dose and dosage regimen based on previous TDM results and obtained therapeutic response.
- Giving expertise for evaluation of data and results for non-compliance, insignificant bioavailability, medication errors, drug interaction etc.
- Assisting the clinician during dose adjustment for patients who are on hemodialysis or peritoneal dialysis.
- Advice and management in poison cases and drug induced toxicities.
- TDM related research activity for cost effectiveness, analytical method development and validation etc.

In addition to the above services pharmacist also contributes in various TDM services like managerial, supportive and financial management of budget. Making, implementation, monitoring and execution of TDM activities, schedule, plan, review, rationalization, patients counselling before, during and after TDM etc.

Medication Errors

A medication error refers as unintentional, preventable episode, event or harm to the patients by improper or inappropriate usage of medication. The medication errors may occur and can be controlled by the health care professional, pharmacist, patient or consumer. It can occur in hospital, pharmacies and at home also. The errors occur can be active error or lateral error. Active errors occur at level of healthcare professionals like physicians, pharmacists, nursing staff etc. The result of active error occurs instantaneously and it includes wrong prescription, inappropriate dispensing etc. Lateral errors are outside the control of healthcare professionals. It includes poor storage conditions, mixing of medicine, inappropriate administration etc. Lateral errors may escape detection but the implications of errors are observable. Medication error is broadly incidence in which error occur in medication process, regardless harm occurred to patient. Such medication can be related to professional practice, health care product, procedures and system including prescription, communication, compounding, dispensing, distribution, administration, education, monitoring and use. The medication errors caused by health care professionals may be due to look-alike and sound-alike in practice. The medication errors can occur at any time, from prescription to consumption by the patient.

The term medication error is always confused with other associated terms like medical errors, adverse drug events. Medical error is all the adverse health conditions as a result of personal errors. The person involved in medical error may be physician, nursing staff, pharmacist or any other person involved in health care system. Medication error is subset of medical error. Adverse drug events are damage to the patient result from drug usage. Adverse drug event which may not have caused the harm to the patient but have potential to do so. It includes harm caused by drug and harm caused by usage of drug. There may be over usage or under usage of drug leading to adverse drug events. Adverse drug event may result from medication error but not always. There are near misses between harm caused and harm not caused due to adverse drug event. These near misses provide potential data and information. This data and information can be used and helps hospital administration to avoid occurrence of such events in future, reduce the risk and improve the patient's safety.

The U.S. Food and Drug administration has given advice that, when a prescription is obtained every individual in health care management chain should read it for:

- ***The right medicine:*** The name of medicine and appearance should be checked. The name look-alike and spell-alike creates confusion and errors may occur.
- ***The right patient:*** The name of patient must be checked. Busy pharmacy may dispense the medicine to wrong patients.
- ***The right amount:*** The strength of medicine dispensed should be of correct strength. Over reading of decimal point may leads to dispensing of tenfold less or more dose.
- ***The right time:*** When and how the medicament is taken must be clearly mentioned and told to the patient.
- ***The right route:*** The right route of administration of dosage form should be indicated. Patient may swallow a chewable tablet if not indicated properly.

In 1989 American Society of Health System Pharmacists (ASHP) define medication errors as "Any preventable event that may cause or leads to inappropriate medication use or patients harm while the medication is in control of the health care professional, patient or consumer". The ASHP also define the causes of medication error incorporation. It involves prescription errors, dispensing medication errors, administration errors and patient's compliance errors.

Prescription Errors

A prescriber makes unintentional error during prescribing. The poor handwriting may be one of the potential reasons for prescription error. Prescription errors may go unidentified because other healthcare professional misinterpret it. Prescription errors consist of prescribing errors, incorrect selection of drug, omission errors, wrong time, improper dose (higher or lesser), wrong dosage form, wrong selection of patients, illegible handwriting, directional errors etc. The physicians are no longer held solely responsible for prescription errors. Pharmacist, nursing staff can contribute in correction of medication errors in prescriptions. Various ways by which prescription errors can be minimized includes:

- Use of formulary system during prescribing the drugs. The guidelines given in formulary system will help the physician to prescribe error free.
- Patients should make sure that doctors should know every medicine he is taking. Many time patients take over-the-counter medicine, dietary supplements such as vitamins, herbal products, along with prescription medicine which can become a potential cause for medication error.
- During visit to the doctor, patient should bring and show all the medicines to physician. Doctors can see and help patients if there any problem. Doctors can keep and update their record of the medicine consumed by patient.
- Patients should see that doctor should know about any kind of allergy or adverse reaction he has had to the specific drug, substance if any.
- Patient should make sure that he can read the prescription and instruction written in by doctor. If patient cannot read it pharmacist should help him to understand the instruction.

- Patient should ask for the information about medicine prescribed to him. The information about what for medicine, how to take medicine, likely side effects, safety of medicine, dietary supplement needed or to be avoided etc.

Dispensing Medication Errors

Dispensing is carried out in hospital or medical shop. The common dispensing error is selection of wrong product. Selection of wrong product may occur due unintentional errors like look-alike, spell-alike product. Spelling mistake or ineligible handwriting of prescriber may be a leading cause of dispensing medication errors. Other cause of dispensing medication errors includes miscalculation, wrong dose sent, dose borrowed from another patient, heavy workload and busy pharmacist. Various ways by which dispensing medication errors can be minimized includes:

- Patient should ask pharmacist instructions regarding how to take medicine.
- When patient picks up medicine he should confirm that the medicine is same the doctor have prescribed.
- Patient should read the instructions given on the label if any and understand it. Any clarification or further information needed can be obtained from the pharmacist.
- Pharmacist can help patient in using household techniques in measuring the liquid medicine. Like use of closure of container or defining size of spoon etc.
- Pharmacist should make aware the patient regarding side effects if any. Anti-allergic medicine containing antihistaminic cause's drowsiness. The patient should be made aware regarding this side effect and should not drive vehicle or operate heavy machines.

Administration Errors

A very little is documented regarding errors that occur during administration. The errors in administration include omission of drug, failure to check identity of patient, improper administration techniques, use of wrong and expired medicine, selection of wrong route for drug administration etc. Deliberate violation of instruction and guidelines given by physician, pharmacist or written on prescription and label of the medicine, during administration of medicine is one of the potential cause of administration error.

- Patient should learn about medicine. He should clearly understand from doctor or pharmacist regarding treatment plan, drug administration schedule, dose of drug, special precaution to be taken if any etc.
- Patients should always speak up if he/she has question in mind. Patients have right to ask the question regarding treatment he/she is taking.
- Patients should take the correct medicine timely in correct dose as asked to do so by physician or pharmacist. He should not make any deviation in dosing, frequency, time of administration of himself. This may leads to overdosing or under dosing. In both the cases patient will be in dangerous situation.
- Patients can use color code, proper labeling for taking medicine.
- If patient has many health problems he should look that some primary health care professional is there to look after his care.
- Patients should take care that all the health care professionals attending him has all the information regarding his illness? Patient should not assume that everyone knows about his illness.

Role of Pharmacist

Pharmacist is expected to play important and pivotal role in reducing the medication errors and misuse. Intervention of pharmacist in preventing medication errors has lead to proper documentation of medication errors and measures can be taken for their reduction and prevention. Pharmacist should work collaboratively with physician and other health care professionals in developing, implementing and monitoring therapeutic plans to produce appropriate therapeutic efficacy in patients. Pharmacist can contribute for reduction of medication errors at all levels where these errors occur like prescribing, dispensing and administration. In his own job of dispensing pharmacist should ensure that errors will not occur at any point in dispensing process. The suggested recommendations for pharmacist are as follows.

- Pharmacist should bring the medication errors and mistakes in prescriptions to the notice of prescriber in professional manner playing the complementary and supportive role.
- Pharmacist should participate in drug therapy monitoring, assessment of therapeutic appropriateness, medication administration appropriateness, duplication of therapy, possible interaction review etc. Pharmacist should also participate in other activity which will help to achieve safe, effective, rational use of drugs.
- Pharmacists recognize and recommend appropriate drug therapy. He should update himself with current knowledge of therapeutics through literature, consultation with other healthcare professionals. He should participate in continuing education programs for knowledge update.
- Pharmacist should make themselves available round the clock for healthcare professionals, patients to offer the information and advice he can contribute in drug therapeutic and rational use of medicine.
- Pharmacist should be well aware about the prescription and medication ordering system, drug distribution policy and procedures established by the hospital administration. He should find out the loopholes, might be responsible for medication errors and should take a proper measure for their prevention.
- Pharmacist should not assume, guess during dispensing of confusing prescriptions. Any query should be referred back to the prescriber for necessary correction or clarification.
- During dispensing pharmacist should maintain the order of dispensing and cleanliness in working area. During dispensing, Good Dispensing Practice should be followed. One procedure should be performed at a time.
- The original copy of prescription should be reviewed before dispensing. All the work should be done with appropriate supportive persons using automated devices and machinery. All the procedures to be followed must be confirmed and executed. Pharmacist should have minimal participation and interference in self checking the process of dispensing. During high risk dispensing all the work procedure must be checked by second authorized individual.

- Whenever possible the medicine must be dispensed in ready to administered form. No any secondary procedures like dilution, addition of components should be handed over to the patient's part. Unit dose dispensing should be preferred for drug distribution.
- The labels should be used cautiously to convey clear message to the patient like "shake well before use," "for external use only," "not for injection" etc.
- The medicine should be dispensed to the patients timely and as per the policy of the hospital.
- By using his counseling skill pharmacist should observe how the medicines are administered and utilized. He should also ensure regarding appropriate usage, proper storage of the medicine.
- Pharmacist should take a review of medicines which are returned back. Such returned medicine gives an idea about how many amount of medicine has been administered by the patients and how much number of dosages has been missed.
- Pharmacist should counsel the ambulatory patients during dispensing of medications. Pharmacist should verify why these medicines are prescribed for patients. The message should be conveyed to the patients in his language about importance of drug administration, in timely, accurate dose and as per instructions.
- Pharmacist should advice to the patients regarding contents and medication orders, precautions printed in the leaflet available with medicine.
- Pharmacist should keep the record of dispensed medicine and details of the patients for tracking the information at other time.

References

20 Tips to help prevent medical errors, Agency for healthcare research and quality, www.ahrq.gov.

A Program Guide For Public Health, Partnering with Pharmacists in the Prevention and Control of Chronic Diseases, National Center for Chronic Disease Prevention and Health Promotion.

A.J. Winfield, R.M.E. Richards (2004). Pharmaceutical Practice, 3rd edition, Churchill Livingstone.

A.M. Ageel, Drug and poison information centre in the college of pharmacy, University of Riyad.

Academy of Managed Care Pharmacy, American Medical Association, American Society of Health-System Pharmacists, Department of Veterans Affairs, National Business Coalition on Health, U.S. Pharmacopeia, Principles of a Sound Drug Formulary System.

American Society of Hospital Pharmacists (1993). ASHP guidelines on preventing medication errors in hospitals. *Am J Hosp Pharm.* **50:** 305-314.

Christopher W. James (2006). The hospital pharmacist as a partner in healthcare for patients with HIV infection. *Adv Stud Pharm* **3(5):** 172-178.

Cooper and Gunn (1987). Dispensing for Pharmaceutical Students, 12th edition, CBS publishers.

David Jones (2009). Therapeutic drug monitoring - a vital pharmacy role. *The British Journal of Clinical Pharmacy* **1:** 171.

DJP Williams (2007). Medication errors. *J R Coll Physicians Edinb.* **37:** 343-346.

Drug and Therapeutic committee - A practical guide, World Health Organization (2003).

Drug and therapeutic committee training course, Session 1, Drug and therapeutic committee - overview, Participants guide, USAID from the American people, World Health Organization, management science for health.

G. Parthasarathi, Karin Nyfort-Hansen, Milap C Nahata (2012). A Textbook of Clinical Pharmacy Practice, Essential Concepts and Skills, 2nd edition, Universities Press (India) Private Limited.

Indian Public Health standards (IHPS) for primary health centers, Guidelines (March 2006), Directorate General of health Services, Ministry of health and Family Welfare, Govt. of India.

Jozef Novotny, Tomas Eech, The therapeutic drug monitoring as a basis for individualizing patient dosage regimen, *Journal of Health Sciences Management and Public Health* 42-57.

K.G. Ravikumar, B.D. Miglani (2009). A Textbook of Pharmacy Practice; 1st edition, Career Publications.

Karin Wiedenmayer, Rob S. Summers, Clare A. Mackie, Andries G. S. Gous, Marthe Everard, Dick Tromp (2006). Developing Pharmacy Practice - A focus on patient care, handbook, World Health Organization in collaboration with Indian Pharmaceutical federation.

N.K. Jain, S.N. Sharma (1997). A text book of Professional Pharmacy, 4th edition, Vallabh Prakashan, New Delhi.

National Drug Policy for South Africa, 1994.

Niloufar Mohammadpour, Sepideh Elyasi, Naser Vahdati, Amir Hooshang Mohammadpour, Jamal Shamsara (2011). A Review on Therapeutic Drug Monitoring of Immunosuppressant Drugs. *Iranian Journal of Basic Medical Sciences* **14(6):** 485-498.

Office Memorandum, Department of health and family welfare, Ministry of family and welfare, Government of India, dt. 13 Sept. 2010.

Patients safety: preventing medical errors, Self-learning packet (2004), Orlando Regional Healthcare, Education & Development.

Peter Stuchbery, David CM. Kong, Giovanna N. Desantis, Sung K. Lo. (2007). Identification by observation of clinical pharmacists' activities in a hospital inpatient setting. *Pharmacy Practice* **5(1):** 10-16.

R. F. Bridgman, M. I. Roemer (1973). Hospital legislation and hospital system, World Health Organization.

Remington (2005). The Science &Practice of Pharmacy, 21st ed, Lippincott Williams & Wilkins.

Sheena Williamson (2009). Reporting medication errors and near misses, medication safety: An essential guide, Molly Courtenay and Matt Griffiths, Cambridge University Press, 155-171.

Shobha C, Ramesh M, Parthasarathi G (2011). Poison information centre–An overview of its significance, organization and functioning. *Indian Journal of Pharmacy Practice* **4(4):** 14-20.

Tobias Mettler and Peter Rohner (2009). E-Procurement in Hospital Pharmacies: An Exploratory Multi-Case Study from Switzerland. *Journal of Theoretical and Applied Electronic Commerce Research* **4(1):** 23-38.

www.pfizer.com/medicinesafety

CHAPTER 5

Adverse Drug Reactions

Definition

Administration of medicine provided benefits to the society. Use of medicaments is unquestionable. It has reduced the mortality rate. Vaccination, treatment and preventive measures have reduced the child illness, abnormality and mortality. The drugs and medicaments are administered for prevention, diagnosis, cure of diseases. These medicines are from various sources like drugs, biological, diagnostics, natural and nutritional supplements etc.

Along with their therapeutic effects these administered drug also elucidate other effects termed as side effects, untoward effects, adverse effects, toxic effects etc. depending on the severity of these effects. Most of the time these other effects are known or predictable. Some of the time they are unknown and their occurrence cannot be predicted. The occurrence of such effect is also depends on individual person and drugs. The person-to-person variability to the drug response is a major contributing factor in clinical practice. This leads to therapeutic failure, adverse drug reactions in individual patients or subpopulation of patients.

Side effect: It is unintended effect either beneficial or adverse occurred due to a drug or dosage form at the dose normally administered. The side effect is related to pharmacological property of a drug and does not required termination or stoppage of treatment. For example, dryness of mouth during anticholinergic treatment.

Adverse drug effect: It is untoward effect of a drug or dosage form that is present during treatment along with therapeutic effect. Adverse effects are more serious than side effects and require special attention, stopping the treatment or alteration in the treatment. For example, minor allergic reaction to a certain category of drugs.

Adverse Drug Events (ADE): It is unwanted occurrence of event, fatal action, injury or medical occurrence during or after treatment with medicine or other aids. ADE are caused by effect of use of drugs like side effect, adverse effect etc. or harm from the use of drug like dose reduction, discontinuation of drug therapy etc. It does not have casual relationship with treatment.

Serious adverse effect: It is a life threatening fatal effect of the drug administration. Requires prolonged hospital admission or its occurrence. It may leads to persistence disability or incapability. For example, anaphylactic reactions.

Adverse Drug Reactions (ADR): It is unexpected, undesirable effect of drug or dosage form when administered in therapeutic range and requires immediate stoppage of treatment or selection of alternate drug. According to World Health Organization, ADR is described as "A response to a drug that is noxious and unintended, and that occurs at doses normally used in humans for the prophylaxis, diagnosis or therapy of disease or for the modification of physiological function". This definition does not include the fact of therapeutic failure of drug and drug abuse, overdose and poisoning of drugs. It is independent of mechanism of ADR, allergies, idiosyncrasies, pharmacological and toxicological mechanism and interaction between different drug and food (drug and food interaction). Karch and Lasagna defined ADR as "Any response to a drug that is noxious and unintended, and that occurs at dosage used in human for prophylaxis, diagnosis, or therapy, excluding failure to accomplish the intended purpose". As per Food and Drug Administration, for reporting purpose ADR is defined as "Event related to drugs or device in which patients outcome is death, life-threatening, real risk of dying, hospitalization, (initial or prolonged), disability which may be significant, persistent or permanent, congenital anomaly, or require intervention to prevent permanent impairment or damage. Laurence's definite ADR as "A harmful or significantly unpleasant effect caused by a drug at doses intended for therapeutic effect or prophylaxis or diagnosis, which warrants reduction of dose or withdrawal of the drug and/or foretells hazard from future administration". It excludes minor unwanted effects like dryness of mouth.

As per the American Society of Hospital Pharmacists (ASHP) ADR is unexpected, unintended, undesired, or excessive response to drug that requires discontinuation of therapy, change of drug therapy, modification of dose, minor adjustment of dose, admission to hospital, prolonged stay in health care facility, needs supportive treatment, have complicated diagnosis, negatively affects prognosis and that leads to temporary or permanent harm, disability or even death of patient. Edwards and Aronson, in 2000 define ADR as "An appreciably harmful or unpleasant reaction, resulting from an intervention related to the use of a medicinal product, which predicts hazard from future administration and warrants prevention or specific treatment, or alteration of the dosage regimen or withdrawal of the product".

ADR is associated with significant morbidity and mortality in hospitalized patients. It is considered to be a 5th leading cause of death amongst them. ADR occurs in 10 to 20% of hospitalized patients. ADR accounts for 5 to 10% cost of hospital admission. Hence in addition to morbidity and mortality it imposes economic burden of health care system and prolongs hospital stay and increases cost of treatment. The biggest tragedy of ADR occurs in 1960s known as **thalidomide tragedy**. There after the need and interest in ADR monitoring, reporting were taken into account. The systematic studies were carried out and strategies were planned, implemented and monitored for avoiding ADRs. In Indian contest around 6% admissions in emergency department are due to ADR.

The term ADR and adverse effects are used interchangeably. Very thin difference separates them from each other. ADR is seen from patient's point of view where as adverse effect is seen from drugs point of view. The term ADR and ADE must be clearly distinguished. Many times they are used interchangeably or as synonymous. ADR is intrinsic property of drug and cannot be avoided. ADR has direct relation with treatment of drug whereas ADE is fatal effect result from medical intervention related to drugs and it includes ADR. ADE has casual relationship with treatment. Drug is one of the contributory causes of ADE. India has become a member of WHO-ADR monitoring program. The pattern of drug usage and ADR in India is quite different due to diversity in socioeconomic status, ethical, nutritional and other factors. The Drug Controller General of India (DCGI) and Indian Council of Medical Research (ICMR) has established ADR monitoring centers in many hospitals in India. Still the pharmacovigilance is in infant stage. Lack of public awareness, deficiency of staff in health care chain is major contributors for poor pharmacovigilance about ADR.

Factors Affecting ADR

The ADR is counter part of therapeutic effect of drug administered for various purposes like diagnosis, treatment, mitigation etc. The therapeutic effect for drug depends on various factors and so ADR also. The factors that contributes the ADR includes:

Age

Pediatric patients have immature hepatic function, with hepatic microsomal enzyme system is immature state. Where as in geriatric patients the hepatic function is abnormal. Hepatic microsomal system is weak in geriatric patients. This immature and abnormal hepatic function may accounts for inappropriate metabolism of drug administered and accounts for ADR. Incidences of ADR increases with age due to change in pharmacokinetics and pharmacodynamics associated with age. Pediatric patients has reduced rate of clearance and may encounter for ADR. A well known example of pediatric ADR is gray baby syndrome associated with chloramphenicol.

Gender

Females are more prone to ADR as compared to males. The relative body surface area and size of females is smaller than males. The hormonal status of females is significantly changing as compared to males. The fat distribution is also different and accounts for difference in pharmacokinetics and pharmacodynamics status. This diversified pharmacokinetics and pharmacodynamics accounts for difference in

ADR. Females undergo regular hormonal changes during menstrual cycle, pregnancy and lactation. These phases must be considered during ADR.

Co-administration of Drugs

Co-administration of drugs has direct relationship with ADR. More the number of co-administered drugs, greater will be the change of ADR. Patients taking many drugs simultaneously are at greater risk of ADR.

Route of Administration

Wrong selection of route of administration leads to ADR. Route of administration determines the rate at which drug reaches in systemic circulation. Faster the drug get entry in systemic circulation, smaller will be the dose. If drug is given too quickly *via* intravenous administration, risk of occurrence ADR increases. The problem can be resolved by giving slow intravenous injection or infusion.

Presence of Diseases

Presence of diseases like hepatitis, renal insufficiency, and cardiac complications alters the drug distribution, metabolism and excretion significantly. This may results in accumulation of drug in body and accounts for ADR.

History of ADR

ADR is more frequently encounter in patients who previously suffered from ADR. The patient have allergic tendency and account for ADR significantly.

Patient's Condition

The magnitudes of problem with patient have proportionate relationship with ADR. This is because large number of drugs will be used in critical patients and accounts for more frequent ADR. Geriatric patients, critical care patients and patients undergoing complicated surgical procedures are more prone for ADR.

Life style

A patient's life style also governs ADR. Patients habitual of tobacco chewing, smoking, alcoholism are at greater risk of ADR. These habits contribute for change in hepatic, renal function and leads to ADR.

Genetics

A genetic abnormality also accounts for ADR. Number of genetic polymorphism is present populations. Certain patients with specific genetics may encounter with ADR.

Dose

Dose of drug has direct relationship with ADR. Larger dose drug has high risk ADR as compared to low dose drug. Dose related ADR is mostly of Type A. Reduction of dose reduces incidences of ADR.

Formulation

ADR can also encounter due to presence of excipients present in formulations. The particle size of active pharmaceutical ingredient affects bioavailability and enhanced bioavailability may leads to ADR. Best example for formulation related ADR is substitution of diluents calcium sulphate with lactose in phenytoin formulation leading to toxicity.

The class of drug also determines the occurrence of ADR. Some classes cause frequent ADR while others are comparatively safe. The classes of drugs like antibiotics, anticancer are more prone to ADR. Drugs from CNS category are safer. Depending on order of severity and frequency of ADR occurrence in different category of drug is antibiotics > antitumor agents > anticoagulants > cardiovascular agents > anticonvulsants > anti diabetics > antihypertensive > analgesics > antiasthmatics > sedatives and hypnotics > antidepressants > antipsychotics > drugs used in peptic ulcers. Similarly some responses occasionally occur as ADR while others are not. The frequency of occurrence of effects as ADR is bone marrow suppression > bleeding > CNS > allergic/skin > metabolic > cardiac > GIT > renal > respiratory. More than 16% patients suffer from bone marrow suppression while respiratory related ADR were found in very rare patients.

Significance of ADR in Health Care System

India has emerged as a hub for clinical trials due to its large, diversified population and availability of patients suffering from diseases like diabetes, cancer and cardiovascular complications. For clinical trials, India offers around 700000 specialized hospital beds. India is fourth leading country producing pharmaceuticals worldwide. More than 6000 licenses pharmaceutical companies manufacturing around 60,000 brands exist in India. Many of new drugs are introduced in Indian market. India is also a largest hub for herbal and traditional medicines. It is believed that herbal medicines are safe. However these medicines are adulterated with allopathic medicines like steroids to present efficacy. Many such incidences have been reported in past. Hence there is immense need of consideration and monitoring of ADR.

Cost is involved in every aspect of health care system. ADR also involves cost. Hence ADR must be considered one of the important contributing factors in health care system chain. The chances of reoccurrence of ADR is very high if it is poorly documented or non-reported. The establishment of reporting and documenting system for ADR involved heavy cost. In India only 1% ADR was reported as compared to 5% worldwide and to overcome this gap pharmacovigilance was established by Ministry of Health and Family Welfare, Govt. of India. The purpose of this cell is to collect and analyze the ADR data. Major Indian population prefers the Govt. hospital for their health care management and hence these hospitals can be a potential source for this type of data.

ADR causes morbidity and mortality. It involves additional cost in treatment of ADR which is over and above to the main course treatment of illness. ADR events occur in every hospital but almost daily in medium size hospitals and outpatient centers. Unnecessary hospitalization due to ADR leads to loss of health as well as quality of life and waste of money. It means unnecessary hospitalization due to ADR is very inefficient. Prevention will avoid this wastage of health and money. Hence prevention of ADR should be a prime goal of health care management system.

Classification of ADR

ADR can be classified depending on mechanism they work. It is classified as Type A or Type B. ADR of Type A is pharmacological ADR. ADR of Type B involves idiosyncratic reactions. This classification was based on involvement of immunological reactions. Type A reaction does not involves immunological reactions while Type B reaction involves immunological reactions. According to Rawlins and Thompson classification, Type A reaction does not involves immunological reaction. It is over enhancement of therapeutic response. Type B reactions are due to immunological responses. Few authors have also indicated Type C and Type D reaction. Type C reactions are associated with prolonged therapy like nephrotoxicity associated with prolonged use of analgesics. Type D reaction consists of delayed reactions like carcinogenicity or teratogenicity.

Type A

Type A includes ADR to the drug that is related to pharmacological response of drug. It is also referred as toxic, side or secondary effect of drug. Pharmacological ADR (Type A) are most common. They occur in around 25 to 45% patients. They are predictable and are dose dependent. The ADR are related to primary and secondary pharmacological response of drug. The factors that affect the ADR includes dose of drug, pharmaceutical variation in formulation, pharmacokinetics, pharmacodynamics, drug-drug interactions. Pharmacological ADR (Type A) occurs when the plasma concentration of drug exceeds the effective therapeutic range or when there is increased sensitivity to the drug. The toxicity occurs in the region where drug elucidates its effect. Examples of such ADR include gastric irritation, hyper acidity or peptic ulceration due to treatment of NSAIDs reaction of gout from treatment of thiazide diuretics, bone marrow suppression followed by treatment of methotrexate.

Type B

Other type of ADR (Type B) is associated with idiosyncratic reactions. Type B reactions are not predictable. Idiosyncratic ADR are less common and non specific. They do not show relationship with dose administered and severity of reaction. Toxicity affects many organs and systems. Type B reactions are also referred as drug intolerance, hypersensitivity etc. The mechanism of type B reaction is not clear, poorly understood and occurs due to abnormal reaction from receptors, abnormality in biological systems, immunological reactions. Type B reactions are host dependent. Example for such reaction includes anaphylactic reaction, allergic reactions to the drugs like penicillin. Type B reactions are further subdivided in various categories depending on mechanism of occurrence of these reactions.

Type I (Anaphylactic reaction): This is also known as hypersensitivity reaction. This is one of the most common amongst Type B reactions. This ADR is most common for certain category of drugs like penicillin. The individual patients are more sensitive for Type I reactions. Type I reaction occurs typically after second or third exposure to the drug. The reactions occur even when a very small amount is administered by any route of administration. The signs and symptoms are dramatic, rapid and prompt. Immediate treatment is requiring for prevention of complication from type I reactions. The mechanism involves recognition of drug molecule by IgE on the surface of mast cells and subsequently release of substances like histamine, inflammatory mediators leading to degranulation of cells.

Type II (Antibody mediated): This type of reaction occurs between drug and protein molecules (antibody) on cell membrane or circulating. The circulating antibodies like IgG, IgM form complexation with drug and leads to activation. The affected system by this reaction is hematological system. The most common outcome of this reactions are hemolytic anemia, thrombocytopenia, agranulocytosis etc.

Type III (Immune reactions): Type III reaction occurs as a result of administration of foreign serum or serum product to the patients. It also occurs with certain drugs like penicillin, streptomycin etc. There is formation of antigen-antibody complex leading to lodging of capillary blood vessels of vital organs like skin, kidney, liver etc. leading to lupus erythematosus. The signs and symptoms include fever, urticaria, protein urea, eosinophilia etc.

Type IV (Cell mediate reaction): A typical example of Type IV reaction is contact dermatitis produced by application of certain drugs or substances to skin. It is due to formation of complex with proteins which triggers lymphatic cellular immune reaction.

Pseudoallergic reaction: These reactions occur due to similar category of drug mentioned in above Type I, II, III and IV reactions. It does not involve immune system directly. The substances release immunological mediators by some other mechanism. This reaction occurs even after first exposure to the molecule rather than previous sensitization after 2 to 3 administrations. The typical reaction includes itching, bronchospasm, flushing, urticaria or even circulatory shock.

	Type A	**Type B**
Termed as	Predictable, side effect, toxic effect, augmented, dose related	Unpredictable, allergic reaction, idiosyncratic, intolerance, qualitative, dose-independent, bizarre
Mechanism	Predictable, understood, same as that of drug	Poorly understood, indifferent
Incidences	High	Low
Morbidity	Mild	Sever
Mortality	Low	High
Frequency	Reproducible and common	Non reproducible and uncommon
Detection	Fast – during Phase 1 to 3 of clinical trial	Rare – mostly during Phase 4 of clinical trial
Treatment	Same as drug poisoning	Stop treatment, symptomatic
Severity	Variable but mild	Variable but more severe
Cause	Overdose of drug	Hypersensitivity to drug
Dose	Good relation with dose. Occurs with more than therapeutics	No simple relationship with dose. Occur at any dose (even low than therapeutic dose)
Predictability	Yes	No
Management	Dose reduction	Drug withdrawal
Example	Gastric irritation, hypoglycemia, lowering of blood pressure	Anaphylactic reactions, allergic reactions etc.
Proportion	80%	20%
Animal model	Usually reproduced	No known model available

ADR reaction type	Drug	Toxicity	Reaction/Mechanism
Type A			
Pharmaceutical	Phenytoin	Ataxia, nystagmus	Increases bioavailability due to change in formulation
Pharmacokinetic	Digoxin	Nausea, arrhythmia	Increased elimination if renal function is impaired
Pharmacodynamic	Indomethacin	Left ventricular failure	Water and sodium retention.
Genetic	Nortriptyline	Confusion	Reduced hepatic elimination due to deficiency of CYP2D6
Drug interaction	Lithium and NSAIDs	Lithium toxicity	Inhibition of lithium excretion
Type B*			
Generalized reaction	Penicillin	Anaphylaxis	
Generalized reaction	Temafloxacin	Hypersensitivity	
Skin	NSAIDs	Epidermal necrosis	
Liver	Halothane	Hepatitis	
Homological system	Remoxipride Clozapine Nomifensine	Aplastic anemia Agranulocytosis Haemolysis	
CNS	Zimeldine	Guillain-Barre syndrome	
Kidney	Penicillin	Interstitial nephritis	
Lungs	Dapsone	Pneumonitis	
Heart	Tacrolimus	Cardiomyopathy	
Reproductive	Etretinate	Foetal abnormalities	

* NOTE: Reaction mechanism is not required here

Causality of ADR

ADR leads to morbidity and mortality. It is a leading cause of death amongst hospitalized patients. ADR also contributes for elevation of treatment cost. If not handled or treated properly it leads to a causality. Thalidomide tragedy is amongst biggest example of ADR. Thalidomide was prescribed to thousand of pregnant woman causing severe form of limb abnormalities. That was the even led to development of modern drug regulation and confirms the need of ADR. It gives the understanding that ADR of drug might be beyond the anticipation of therapeutic effect during clinical practice. Now a day, monitoring system and proper care of patients decline the incidences of ADR. The events that occur are mild and disappear when dose is reduced or drug is stopped. Sometime ADR might be serious and long lasting.

When ADR is suspected, it might be helpful to assess how likely it will occur due to medicine. The factors that are responsible for causality due to ADR include nature of reaction, timing, dose relationship. Some clinical symptoms occurs occasionally includes skin reactions. Such incidences were caused by medicine. The duration from administration of drug to the occurrence of ADR is the characteristic of ADR reaction occurred. Anaphylactic reaction develops within few minutes, on other hand some reaction take months to years to develop. Some reaction may be developed in next generation. Administration of diethylstilbestrol by a pregnant woman leads to a vaginal cancer in her girl child. Most of the time, dose ADR relationship is linear. Reduction of dose reduces incidences of ADR. If ADR resolved on stoppage of drug and recur after administration indicates that medicine is responsible for ADR. The overlapping symptoms of illness and ADR reaction due to drug-drug or drug-food interaction must be taken in account.

In the view of above discussion it becomes essential to establish a relationship of causality with ADR. The occurrence of ADR should be assessed on probability scale. Many methods have been proposed and established to assess the causality ADR relationship. The methods range from short questionnaire to the statistical algorithms. Establishments of this relation will help in preventing further occurrence of ADR. These probability scales should be structured, transparent, consistent and easy to apply.

Number of methods of causality assessment have been published by different authors. More than thirty four different methods have been proposed. These methods can be categorized in three classes: expert judgments, algorithm and probabilistic methods. Expert judgment based on individual knowledge and experience to handle the causality of ADR. Algorithms are set of questionnaire, and include calculation of score depending on answers to these questions. Probabilistic method use specific finding of previously established probability in estimating posterior probability calculations. No single method was universally accepted. Different category of causality was estimated using different methods. The causality assessment system proposed by World Health Organization for International Drug Monitoring, Uppsala Monitoring Centre (WHO-UMC) is generally accepted scale and most widely used method for causality assessment in clinical practice.

Pharmacovigilance

Clinical trials for the new drug were carried out in small number of peoples before licensing. Children's and geriatric patients are mostly omitted from clinical trials and hence lack the supporting data and evidences for alteration in anatomical, physiological, pathological or biochemical parameters. In clinical practice millions of pediatric and geriatric patients are included. Along with that the patients might have adult individual which have different biological parameters from representative in clinical trials.

The clinical trials are carried out in very strict, ideal and stringent condition. On contrast the medicine used in clinical practice suffers much diversity. The medicines are not used in controlled environment. There might be difference in pharmacokinetics and pharmacodynamics in patients taking these medicines. The individual patients might suffer from same illness but differ from each other in respect of ADR. The clinical trial identifies most of the therapeutic aspects; common and predictable side effect of the medicine, but might fails to pinpoint the occurrence of ADR. The rare side effects and ADR might be seen once when medicine is used in large population of patients. The representative data in group of peoples can give idea about ADR but could not give complete emphasis so that ADR can be avoided. Hence post marketing surveillance get importance along with pharmacovigilance of the drug.

Important risk factor in development of ADR is re-exposure and poor documentation of evidenced if occurred in previous administration. This leads to experience of same ADR again and again. This emphasizes the documentation of ADR. Pharmacovigilance is detection, monitoring, reporting, assessment and prevention of ADR. ADR can occur in any therapeutic regimen. Multiple drug therapy, increased age, pediatric patients, co-morbid diseases are the contributing factors which increases the chance of occurrence of ADR. Poor reporting, lack of awareness, ignorance of symptoms results in inadequate ADR monitoring. Implementation of effective pharmacovigilance programs is need of time as the India is country with wide genetic diversity.

As per the WHO, "Pharmacovigilance is the science and activities relating to the detection, assessment, understanding and prevention of adverse effects or any other medicine related problem". Various countries have established pharmacovigilance centers for monitoring and reporting of ADR.

Objectives: The important objectives of pharmacovigilance include:

- To improve patients care and safety in respect of medicinal use including other medical and paramedical interventions.
- To improve in public health and safety related to medicinal use.
- To detect the problems related to use of medicine and timely communication of outcome.
- To Assess of benefits, harms, effectiveness and risk of irrational use of medicine.
- To encourage safe, rational, effective and cost effective use of medicines.
- To promote, understanding, education and training in pharmacovigilance and its effective percolation in personals involved in health care system and public.
- To collect and manage the ADR data for safe use of medicine and evaluation of this data for decision making with respect to safe use of medicine.

Detection: Detection of ADR from illness become difficult most of the time since both ADR and illness might act through the same physiological and pathological pathway. Implementation of few approaches might helpful in detecting ADR.

- Medical practitioner should confirm that medicine ordered are same the medicine received and medicine administered by the patient in the recommended dose.
- Appropriate history taking and patient's examination must be done before treating illness. Recording full medical history and examination of patient for illness (with supporting laboratory, pathological examination if required) will help in guessing the possible ADR.
- ADR reaction occurs instantly or delayed. Detecting them by simple counseling questions will help to avoid them.
- Effect of withdrawal of medicine and re-introduction of medicine after withdrawal should be determined.
- Medical practitioner must know the pharmacology of medicine. He should check the suspected reaction reported if any, in books or package inserts. It must be remembered that even if the reaction is not documented in package insert, it does not means reaction cannot occur.

Detection of ADR is a part of patient's diagnosis. Differential diagnosis is required if patient is taking medicine. First it should be investigated that whether patient is taking any over-the-counter medicine that might not be a part of prescription. This may contain herbal preparation, traditional medicinal remedies, dietary supplements, recreational drug, abused drugs etc. The next part will be whether the ADR is due to medicine. If patient is taking several medicines at a time detecting the ADR medicine become difficult and problem become complex. The time and ADR occurrence relationship must be assessed. When the ADR get worst and when the reaction get abate. Does it have relationship with time of drug administration?

The pattern of ADR might fit with known in pattern of pharmacological or allergic reactions of drug. This pattern might have similarity with pathogenesis of disease. This information must not be with new drug even if it is predictable from pharmacological response. The background frequency must be considered, including events and how often it occurs.

Monitoring: Monitoring is the process of checking a system, that changes with time. ADR occurs retrospectively and always requires active monitoring. This is because we do not realize its occurrence till it occurs. The reason behind occurrence is not known. Thus monitoring of ADR becomes limited. A careful attention must be paid during monitoring to note the ADR. Occurrence of ADR with illness makes it difficult for medical practitioner to manage the pharmacotherapy and cost of the treatment. The retrospective or concurrent management of regular pharmacotherapy for illness and for ADR cannot be overemphasized. The ADR is the indication to the medical professional regarding something going very wrong.

Prospective monitoring of ADR is always preferred. By this way the ADR can be minimized or can be prevented from occurrence and cost of ADR treatment can be avoided. The prospective monitoring can be managed in series of serious or unusual reaction that sign the occurrence of ADR. The pharmacist has opportunity by patients monitoring that can foreseen and the ADR and can be avoided.

For the effective monitoring of ADR all health care professional must be trained on importance and benefits of ADR reporting. They should be encouraged to report any ADR suspected or observed to the pharmacist or medical practitioner. ADR report should be given high priority for assessment. The ADR reporting procedure and forms must be simplified and easily accessible. ADR reporting program should be always ongoing and respect the patient's confidentiality.

Reporting: Reporting of ADR is must be done to the authorized reporting centers. These reporting centers collect the data, analyze and assess the risk factors associated with it. These legal authorities will be responsible for the management of ADR data. The reporting of ADR data should be done by various non-government agencies, hospital administrations, pharmacies and pharmaceutical companies who are conducting clinical, pre-clinical and post-clinical trials.

- When detected, ADR must be communicated to the health care provider, pharmacies or pharmaceutical company who manufactured it. The information thus obtained by them should be communicated to the suitable health authorities that collect this data. The information must be reported in prescribed format with relevant supporting documents. It is obligatory for pharmaceutical company to provide suitable detail information upon request.
- The ADR from any of the following medical condition after drug administration should be reported
    - Death
    - Life threatening effect
    - Permanent disability
    - Anomaly or birth defect
    - Inpatient hospitalization
    - Prolongation of hospital stay
    - Intervention to prevent permanent impairment
- The ADR information should be reported within specified time frame. The health care provider, pharmacies should submit the ADR within 7 days. The license holder or manufacturer of concerned drug also should be informed about ADR. If complete information is not available at the time of reporting then the follow up documents must be sent within 15 days.
- The monitoring authority should include this information in the product safety reports and update within specified time frame.
- The reporting authorities (health care providers, pharmacies, pharmaceutical companies) should submit ADR information by post, fax or *via* email. Verbal reports will be only accepted in emergency situations and documentation must be completed within specified time frame.
- A prescribed format/form must be used while furnishing the ADR information to the health authority. The minimum information required should include patient's information and identification, details about suspected reaction and suspected drug.

- The additional information of ADR if not available at the time of reporting, should be provided with follow up report. The health authority may delegate a separate agency to collect detail information along with medical record, product information etc. Health care provider, pharmacies, pharmaceutical companies have to comply with the request of health authority.

Safety data collected before phase 4 may not be sufficient to support the products safety profile and ADR. The health authority of country hence imposes to conduct the post marketing surveillance study. Health authority, licensing authority denote this period as post marketing safety monitoring period. During this period pharmaceutical company should proactively collect the safety data, prepare a report periodically and submit them to health authority timely. These reports will be termed as periodic safety update reports.

Preventing: Health care provider, pharmacies and pharmaceutical companies shall manage and conduct the assessment, prevention and treatment programs for known risks. Investigation on potential risks, follow up on post-marketing surveillance data and issues arise there should ensure patients safety. Health care providers, pharmacies and pharmaceutical companies should work for prevention of ADR.

- ***Health authority:***
    - Health authority and delegate agencies should collect the drug safety information and communicate them to health care providers in safeguard of patients.
    - Health authority should carefully assess the risks associated with the drug. The Risk-benefit balance should be carefully concerned in respect to its therapeutic importance.
    - The health regulatory authorities should assess and evaluate the information received to them. In relation to the therapeutic importance the risk-benefit balance of the drug should be evaluated carefully and drug reassessment should be conducted to improve drug safety data base.
    - Health authority should make an appropriate policy to enhance safe use of medicine and make appropriate planning and

arrangement to support the research and activity in improvement of data and safety information.

- ***Health care provider and Pharmacies:***
  - Health care providers should follow the guidelines given by health care authorities for safe use of drug reported to produce ADR.
  - Health care provider should proactively collect the ADR and related data and create database and guidelines on using such high alert drugs. The ADR information should be promptly forwarded to the health authority.
  - Health care providers should establish an internal mechanism for reviewing and reporting of ADR. The mechanism should be capable to indentify, know the risk and detect the potential of such information.
- ***Pharmaceutical companies:***
  - As a mandatory requirement of pharmacovigilance management, pharmaceutical company should arrange and conduct special training programs annually to all related persons. The training programs should be organized to ensure that all the related individuals are capable of performing their duties of pharmacovigilance activity.
  - A special person should be appointed to look after drug safety affairs. This person will be responsible for establishment and execution of training program on pharmacovigilance. He shall be also responsible for establishment of post marketing surveillance and standard operating procedures.
  - The person in charge of safety issue shall be also responsible for preparation of training material of pharmacovigilance, safety issues.
  - Pharmaceutical company should arrange pre-training for newly recruited staff. For existing staff periodic on-job training, refresher courses, content updating programs must be organized.

- If a training program is executed by person other than in charge of safety affairs or external agency then the person in charge should ensure that training has been completed effectively and written documents must be submitted kept with the person in charge.
- The person in charge shall follow all the regulation and keep record of all training programs.

Role of Pharmacist in ADR

ADR is one of the recognized hazards of pharmacotherapy. ADR might be minor without sequel while other causes permanent disability or even death. The World Health Organization (WHO), Food and Drug Administration (FDA) and The Joint Commission on Accreditation of Healthcare Organization have accepted the importance of ADR and established a mechanism for ADR surveillance. Hospitals are made mandatory to have ongoing drug surveillance for detection and evaluate effect of drug and safe, effective drug utilization. Pharmacist play important role in ADR surveillance activity as a reviewer.

Pharmacist is a key person in health care system and drug therapy. Pharmacist is at ideal position in patient's care and who provide vital information regarding drugs and medicines including therapeutic efficacy, safety. The important part is that patient receives medicine in intended treatment benefit and not experience undesired effect known as ADR. If patients experience ADR pharmacist is in position to take appropriate measure to correct the same in various ways. Pharmacist can report event of ADR. Pharmacist might counsel the patients in reducing the ADR. The pharmacist has access to the patient's information and by its knowledge of drugs, he can contribute in guessing and reporting of ADR.

Pharmacists participate in all stages of health care system where medicines are used including medicine ordering, transcribing, dispensing, administering, monitoring, reporting etc. Through counseling pharmacist make learn the patients importance of timely taking medicines. Participating of pharmacist in ward round help the other medical professionals to understand the drug better. Pharmacist have centralized role in safety contributions in preventing, identification, documentation and reporting of ADR. All the health care professionals along with pharmacist have to play a role in maintaining balance between benefits and risk of medicines. Pharmacist understood clearly that no drug is safe completely and pre-marketing trials and studies are carried out in limited group of individuals. The risks are not fully identified, particularly for recently discovered drugs. Keen observation by pharmacist can avoid incidences of ADR in such cases.

Worldwide the National Drug Monitoring program differs in source of participation of reporting ADR by various health care professionals. In Canada and USA majority of ADR were reported by pharmacist. In the countries like France, Ireland, Malaysia, New Zealand and UK majority of ADR were reported by physicians. The reason for reporting low rate of ADR by pharmacist is that these countries have not recognized pharmacist as a reporting authority and not analyzed adequately. A study conducted by agency for healthcare research and quality (AHRQ) of U.S. Department of Health and Human Services concluded that there is 10% reduction in ADR in hospitalized patients who received medication review, counseling, and telephonic follow-up from hospital pharmacist.

Pharmacist interventions during discharge of patients consist of several parts. The medicinal drug regimens during discharge as compared to regimen during hospitalization were compared and discrepancy can be found out. The patients were analyzed for occurrence of ADR during their hospitalization period and make them aware about reporting such events if found after discharge. The patients were advised for medical adherence, therapeutic importance and side effects. Follow-up through telephonic call can be taken for discrepancy in medication and ADR observations, possible remedies for preventable ADR (Ref.ioi50199.pdf). A study concluded that presence of pharmacist in emergency department provides contribution to ADR reporting. The intervention of pharmacist leads to more reporting as compared to spontaneous reporting.

Pharmacist should work as a leader for development, maintenance and evaluation of ADR programs. They should obtain approval from pharmacy and therapeutic committee for conduct of such programs. A training programs in contend updating and quality improvement for the health care professionals must be organized. The pharmacist should:

- Study and analyze each report of ADR.
- Identify drug and patients at the risk from ADR.
- Develop policy and procedure of monitoring and reporting of ADR.
- Prepare document related to the role and responsibility of each person involved in ADR program.
- Use ADR programs for educational purpose.
- Develop, evaluate and maintain the record of reported ADR.
- Report the ADR to the health authorities like Food and Drug Administration.
- Publish or present the important ADR in the medical community meetings, gatherings or conferences.
- Disseminate the important information regarding ADR.
- Take care not to disclose the identity of patient suffering from ADR.
- Maintain the confidentiality of finding and reports.

References

A.J. Winfield, R.M.E. Richards (2004). Pharmaceutical Practice, 3rd edition, Churchill Livingstone.

Arulmani R, Rajendran SD, Suresh B (2008). Adverse drug reaction monitoring in a secondary care hospital in South India. *Br J Clin Pharm* **65(2):** 210-16.

ASCP Guidelines on detection and reporting adverse drug reactions in long term care environments.

ASHP Guidelines on Adverse Drug Reaction Monitoring and Reporting, 126-128.

Assessing, managing and reporting adverse drug reactions may better equip us to minimize medicines-related harm, Basic pharmacy skills, PHARMACY IN PRACTICE (March 2008), 57-61.

Chinese guidance for good clinical pharmacovigilance practice.

G. Parthasarathi, Karin Nyfort-Hansen, Milap C Nahata (2012). A Textbook of Clinical Pharmacy Practice, Essential Concepts and Skills, 2nd edition, Universities Press (India) Private Limited.

Gandhi T.K, Weingart S.N, Borus J, *et al.,* (2003). Adverse drug events in ambulatory care. *N Engl J Med* **348:** 1556-1564.

Guidelines for Detecting and Reporting Adverse Drug Reactions; Individual Case Safety Reports for healthcare professionals; Egyptian pharmacovigilance center (EPVC) 2010.

H.S. Rehan, K. Vasudev, C.D. Tripathi (2002). Adverse drug reaction monitoring, knowledge, attitude and practice of medical students and prescribers. *The National medical journal of India* **15(1):** 24-26.

Hema N.G, Bhuvana K.B, Sangeetha (2012). Pharmacovigilance- The Extent of Awareness Among the Final Year Students, Interns and Postgraduates in a Government Teaching Hospital, *Journal of Clinical and Diagnostic Research* **6(7):** 1248-1253.

I Ralph Edwards, Jeffrey K Aronson, Adverse drug reactions: definitions, diagnosis, and management, The Lancet, (2000), 356, 1255-1259.

International Drug Monitoring (1969). The role of the hospital. *WHO Tech Rep Ser.* 5-24.

J. J. Coleman, R. E. Ferner, S. J. W. Evans (2006). Monitoring for adverse drug reactions. *Br J Clin Pharmacol* **61(4):** 371-378.

Jeffrey L. Schnipper, Jennifer L. Kirwin, Michael C. Cotugno, Stephanie A. Wahlstrom, Brandon A. Brown, Emily Tarvin, Allen Kachalia, Mark Horng, Christopher L. Roy, Sylvia C. McKean, David W. Bates (2006). Role of pharmacist counseling in preventing adverse drug events after hospitalization. *Arch Intern Med* **166:** 565-571.

Johnson Segun Showande, Fakeye Titilayo Oyelola (2013). The concept of adverse drug reaction reporting: awareness among pharmacy students in a Nigerian university. *Internet Journal of Medical Update* **8(1):** 24-30.

K.G. Ravikumar, B.D. Miglani (2009). A Textbook of Pharmacy Practice, 1st edition, Career Publications.

Karch FE and Lasagna L (1977). Towards the Operational Identification of Adverse Drug Reaction. *Clin Pharmacol Ther* **21:** 247-54.

Kristin C. Oberg (1999). Adverse Drug Reactions. *American Journal of Pharmaceutical Education* **63:** 199-204.

Meena Shrivastava, Ganesh Uchit, Ashish Chakravarti, Gajanan Joshi, Mohini Mahatme, Harshal Chaudhari (2011). Adverse Drug Reactions Reported in Indira Gandhi Government Medical College and Hospital, Nagpur. *J A P I* **59:** 1-4.

Monica Zolezzi and Nirasha Parsotam(2005). Adverse drug reaction reporting in New Zealand: implications for pharmacists. *Ther Clin Risk Manag.* **1(3):** 181-188.

Munir N. Gharaibeh, Howard E. Greenberg, Scott A. Waldman (1998). Adverse Drug Reactions: A Review, *Drug Information Journal* **32:** 323–338.

Palphia SS (1996). Genetic variation in India. *Hum Biol* **68:** 607-28.

Rainu Kaushal, David W. Bates, Chapter 7. The Clinical Pharmacist's Role in Preventing Adverse Drug Events, Agency for healthcare research and quality, U.S. Department of health and human services, (www.hhs.gov).

Remington (2005). The Science &Practice of Pharmacy, 21st ed, Lippincott Williams & Wilkins.

Ronald d. Mann, Elizabeth B. Andrews (2007). Pharmacovigilance, 2nd ed.

S Amarnath, S Jaikumar, S Basalingappa, M Thulasimani, and S Ramaswamy (2013). Pharmacovigilance for Health Care Professional Students. *Research Journal of Pharmaceutical, Biological and Chemical Sciences* **4(1):** 1204-1217.

Schnipper JL, Kirwin JL, Cotugno MC. Role of pharmacist counseling in preventing adverse drug events after hospitalization, Agency for healthcare research and quality. U.S. Department of health and human services, (www.hhs.gov).

Sirisha Kalari, Matthew Dormarunno, Oleg Zvenigorodsky, Aparna Mohan (2011). Pharmacy Student Perceptions of Adverse Event Reporting. *American Journal of Pharmaceutical Education* **75(7):** Article 131.

Sivasankari Venkatachalam, Ramachandra Bhat (2012). ADR Monitoring of NSAIDs among the in-Patients of the Orthopedic Ward in a Tertiary Care Centre: A Prospective Observational Study. *Journal of Clinical and Diagnostic Research* **6(1):** 42-46.

Srinivasan R and Ramya G (2011). Adverse drug reaction – causality assessment, International Journal of research in pharmacy and chemistry **1(3):** 606-612.

Sriram S, Ghasemi A, Ramasamy R, Devi M, Balasubramanian R (2011). Prevalence of ADRs at private tertiary care hospital in south India. *J Res Med Sci.* **16(1):** 16-25.

Surendiran A, Balamurugan N, Gunaseelan K, Akhtar S, Reddy K.S, Adithan C (2010). Adverse drug reaction profile of a cisplatin- based chemotherapy regimen in a tertiary care hospital in India: An evaluative study. *Indian J Pharmacol* **42(1):** 40-43.

Syed Ahmed Zaki (2011). Adverse drug reaction and causality assessment scales. *Lung India* **28(2):** 152-153.

Taofikat B. Agbabiaka, Jelena Savovic, Edzard Ernst (2008). Methods of causality Assessment of Adverse Drug Reactions: A systematic Review. *Drug Safety* **31(1):** 21-37.

Yael Ratz, BSc Pharm, Irene Shafir, BSc Pharm, Sofia Berkovitch, BSc Pharm, Moshe Sharristh, MD, Moshe Jacoby, MD, Eran Kozer, MD, Ahuva Golik, MD, Matitiahu Berkovitch, MD, and Shmuel Bar-Haim, MD (2010). The Importance of the Pharmacist in Reporting, Adverse Drug Reactions in the Emergency, Department, *Journal of Clinical Pharmacology* **50:** 1217-1221.

CHAPTER 6

Drug Interactions

Definition

All the drugs administered in therapy have capacity to produce both benefits and risk which are associated with desirable and undesirable effects of drug. Beneficial and Desired effect (therapeutic action) and undesired effect (toxic effect) of a drug depends on the concentration of drug that reaches at the site where drug elucidate its effect. The concentration that achieved at site of action depends on dose of drug administered and the phase of pharmacokinetic (A.D.M.E.) it undergoes. These pharmacokinetic parameters affect the amount of drug that reach at the site of action. Once the drug reaches at site, it interacts with it and elucidates the therapeutic effect. Many of the times it is essential to administered two or more drug simultaneously in order to treat the multiple diseases (for example, diabetes with hypertension or other, along with drug, nutritional supplement, vitamin preparations or medicine from ayurvedic or homeopathy remedy are prescribed. In such conditions there is a chance that the two drugs will interact with each other lead to drug interaction.

The drug interaction is the modification effect of one drug due to presence of other drug, herbal drug, dietary supplement, food material, drink or some other environmental chemical agent. The modification due to drug interaction is quantitative. The intensity/degree of response is either increased or decreased. Some time it might be qualitative i.e., entirely different response which is not predicted is produced. The outcome of such interaction can be beneficial, reduced effect, undesirable or harmful. The drug interaction can be harmful if interaction causes increase in toxicity of drug may be along with or without significant increment in beneficial effect (for example, a patient taking monoamino oxidase inhibitors (MAOI) experiences hypertensive crises when takes meal, containing high amount of tyramine). The reduction in efficacy can be due to drug interaction. The reduction in efficacy leads to sub-therapeutic effect and patient will be deprived from drug therapy (for example, patients taking tetracycline or quinolones if taken with antacid or meal containing divalent metal ions, leads to complexation and reduced absorption of these antibiotics. Reduced absorption decreases plasma concentration of these drugs and therapeutic efficacy). The precipitation of side effect can be one of the outcomes of drug interaction. Otherwise the side effect is very minor and does not have much importance during treatment (for example, patient stabilized on heparin if take aspirin tablet experience sever hemorrhage).

Patients often receive several or more drugs during therapy. Disorders like cancer, AIDS, tuberculosis requires multiple drug therapy or combination of drugs, which works better to achieve desired therapeutic goal. Patients may also have multiple disorders requiring drugs from different categories like diabetes with hypertension, bronchial asthma with rheumatic arthritis. In such conditions multiple drug therapy is must to treat multiple disease conditions. It will not be a surprise if interaction occurs in such condition. The chances of occurrence of drug interactions in such condition are very high.

Many of the time drug interaction is of no clinical significance, in other situation it might have beneficial effect or unwanted medical event requiring extension of treatment. The degree of interaction varies with concentration of drug produces it. When the magnitude of interaction is large it becomes of clinical significance. The drug with narrow therapeutic index tends to have large degree of interaction with small variation in dose. On other hand the drug with large margin of safety tends to have very small outcomes of drug interaction even after large variation in dose of drug. Some drug interactions are intended to enjoy the therapeutic benefits of such interaction. For example, trimethoprime and sulphamethoxazole act on same biochemical pathway of bacterial enzyme system at different places. The outcome of combination of these two drugs is much greater than the mathematical summation of effect of individual drug.

Although the drug related problems develop unexpectedly, drug interactions can be predicted. Most of the drug interactions are related to the physicochemical and pharmacological properties of drugs. Careful monitoring and study of these properties can give the anticipations of drug interactions. However drug interactions become more complicated when more than two drugs interact simultaneously or two drugs interact in presence of third substance. The magnitude and prediction of such interaction diminishes. More number of drugs patient takes, greater will be the chances of drug interactions. Some studies indicates that if patients are taking 6 to 10 per day then the chances of occurrence of drug interaction is around 7%. If the same patient takes around 16 to 20 drugs then chances of occurrence of drug interaction increases to 40%. Taking double number of drugs increases the chance of drug interaction more than five times.

In some cases drug interaction is problematic and complicated in nature. Instead of interaction between two drugs, interaction occurs between one drug and metabolite of other drug. As a natural tendency only drug concentration in plasma is monitored and no one bother about active or inactive metabolite in systemic circulation. This metabolite might have severe interaction with other drug and leads to consequences. Finding the reason of such interaction is too difficult and troublesome. Carbamazepine is metabolized to carbamazepine-epoxide. This metabolite is pharmacologically active and has a significant interaction with co-administered drug valproate. As such carbamazepine and valproate does not have any drug interaction. But when administered, valproate inhibits the metabolism of carbamazepine-epoxide metabolism and accumulation of this active metabolite occurs in body and prolongs the duration of action of carbamazepine.

Contributing Factors

There are many factors that contribute in response to drug interactions. These factors may be drug related or patients related. The factors that contribute in occurrence, severity of drug interaction includes:

Multiple Effects

Most of the drugs used in pharmacotherapy have effects on more than one physiological system. Amongst all the effects one or two might be major effects responsible for therapeutic efficacy of drug, while others might contributes for side effects. When such two drugs are administered which shares common minor effect, then the concerned minor effect become a major effect and precipitate out. When analyzing the drug interaction it is usual tendency to observe the major effects and minor effects may be ignored. These overlooks secondary, minor to very minor effects might contribute in such drug interactions. Pharmacotherapies of combination of phenothiazine (as antipsychotic), imipramine or amitriptyline (antidepressant), trihexyphenidyl (antiparkinson), antihistaminics are used in many patients. All of these categories of drug has considerable different therapeutic applications but shares a single side effect as anticholinergic action. Combination of any two or more drugs will precipitate the cholinergic side effect and leads to significant anticholinergic effect like dryness of mouth, reduced gastric motility etc.

Multiple Prescriptions

A multiple prescription might leads to significant drug interactions. Many time it become necessary to consult more than one physician, especially in geriatric patients where multiple complications were found. The patient refers more than one specialist (for example, diabetologist and cardiologist, orthopedic and psychiatrics etc). The specialist prescribe medicine unknowing that some other specialist also given another prescription. In such situations the medicine prescribed by one physician might have a potential interaction with another medicine. The problem becomes more serious when both specialists not knowing that patient are referring more than one specialist. For example, family physician might have prescribed antihistaminic for common cold for the same patients who take opioid analgesic (for orthopedic treatment) or anxiolytic drug (for psychological treatment). Such combination of drug leads to excessive depressant effect.

Nonprescription Drugs

A major cause of drug interaction is co-administration of non-prescription drugs with prescription drugs. When physician asked the patients about medication they are taking, patient often neglect the disclosure of co-administration of such nonprescription medicines. The nonprescription medicine includes over the counter (OTC) drugs, herbal formulation or dietary supplements. Many patients are taking nonprescription drug for such a long period of time that they even forgot that they are taking medicine. It becomes integral part of their life. The patients taking preparations like analgesics, laxatives, vitamins/calcium supplements, dietary supplements, herbal preparations etc. does not consider as medicine. This information is missed by the patients during questioning from physician. Physician prefers to ask the question based on signs and symptoms of illness and chance of missing the co-administration of such drug is high. These OTC medicines might have potential drug interaction with prescription drugs.

Many of time patients have habits of taking non-prescription drugs (from their previous experience) along with prescription drugs. These two formulations might share a common ingredient and give rise to risk of excessive response or even toxic effect for the ingredient. Antihistaminic are prescribed by physician for various reasons where as many of the OTC products also contains same ingredients leading to sedative effect. Most of the time patients are unaware about this fact during purchasing of OTC products. The drugs that interacts with OTC products or herbal medicine and there outcome is given in table below.

OTC/Herbal drug	Prescribed drug	Interaction
Ibuprofen	Antihypertensive	Increased blood pressure
Ranitidine, femotidine	Antifungal fluconazole, ketoconazole	Decrease drug absorption and make medicine less effective
Antacid, laxatives	Digoxin, fluconazole, ciprofloxacin	Decrease drug absorption and make medicine less effective
Vitamin E	Warfarin	Increased risk of bleeding
Garlic	Anticoagulants, blood thinners, antihypertensive	Increase blood thinning, decrease blood sugar and blood pressure
Ginseng	Antihypertensive, anticoagulants, antidiabetic agents	Headache, insomnia, heart flutter, decreased blood pressure, increased heart rate

Patient's Compliance

Patient's compliance is must for the effective pharmacotherapy. For the various reasons inappropriate administration of medicine might be a cause of drug interaction. Patients do not take the medicine as per the manner it should be taken or intended by the prescriber. Patient may not have received the instruction properly or if received might not understood properly. This could happen due to communication gap or language barrier. In another situation, particularly in geriatric patients due to more number of medicine and their forgetful nature improper drug administration leads to drug interaction. Several drug administration leads to confusion about the many instructions. Patient's compliance leads to not taking dose of medicine or taking in excess dose. In some situation patients forgot to take medicine (leads to under dose) and in compensation take a double dose next time (leads to overdose).

Drug Abuse

Patients has tendency to abuse the medicine. Continuous use of medicine from old prescription for similar symptomatic illness is occasional. Many time abuses are deliberate and lead to incidences of drug interactions. The category of drugs that are abuse includes antihistaminic, anxiolytics, analgesics, laxatives, amphetamines etc.

Age of Patient

Age is important factor to be considered during systematic study of drug interactions. The risk of drug interaction increases with increased age. Geriatric patients are more prone for drug interaction due to more number of drugs taken by them as compared to adults, forgetful nature and deteriorated health. The age related incidences of drug interactions are also significant in newborns as their enzyme system is not fully developed, metabolic processes are not fully developed, renal and hepatic clearance is also immature.

The study indicates that geriatric patients have at least one chronic illness like diabetes, arthritis, hypertension etc. Renal or hepatic impairment in same patient's leads to inappropriate clearance of drugs used in age related disorders, which significantly leads to alteration of metabolism and clearance of these drugs. Due to inadequate metabolism and clearance drug start accumulating in body and drug interactions are evident.

Genetic Factors and Disease Status

Genetic factor contributes for many of the processes associated with drug pharmacokinetics and pharmacodynamics processes. The unexpected reaction might occur in patients of different genetics for the same drug. Isoniazide is metabolized by acetylation process which is influenced by genetics of the patient. Careful dose adjustment is necessary because some individual metabolize Isoniazide rapidly while other very slowly. Administration of same drug from same formulation in fast metabolizing individual leads to under effect while in slow metabolizing individuals it leads to overdosing (peripheral neuritis as side effect). This elevated dose of Isoniazide inhibits metabolism of many other drugs.

Impaired renal function or hepatic functions have significant effect on therapeutic effect of drug. These conditions affect activity of drug in body. Impaired renal function alters clearance and impaired hepatic function changes metabolic status of the drug. Either of this leads to accumulation of drug or under effect of drug administered. The elevated level of drug is unexpected and contributed for drug interaction. Some drugs are bound to plasma proteins in definite fraction. The dose of drug is decided after consideration of this plasma bound fraction of drug. Disease condition like hypoalbumine leads to excess free drug in plasma and account for drug interaction.

Hepatic and Renal Function

Almost all the drugs are metabolized in liver by various enzymatic systems. Hepatic metabolism is necessary for detoxification and conversion of drug molecule in more polar moiety so that its excretion can be facilitated. During hepatic damage the metabolism of drug lowers and prolongation of therapeutic effect occurs. Although the prolongation of therapeutic effect depends on degree of hepatic damage, recognition of hepatic damage will give idea about elevated drug level in body. Small degree of hepatic damage may not alter the metabolic process significantly so that significant change in drug level is observed. The co-administration of another drug which alters the hepatic microsomal enzyme system will have significant effect on such metabolic process and non-significant low or small degree of hepatic damage give significant drug interaction.

Most of the drugs are excreted after metabolism or as it is. Renal clearance is the determinant of stay of drug inside the body after administration. Patient's renal function should be taken in to account when drug is primarily excreted through kidney. Renal impairment leads to prolongation of therapeutic effect and accumulation of drug in systemic circulation. Since the drug is not excreted at normal pace, administration of additional dose leads to significant elevation of systemic concentration of drug resulting in toxicity. Careful dose adjustment is necessary in renal impaired patients. This elevated systemic level of drug might contribute for drug interaction with co-administered drug.

Alcohol and Smoking

Studies have indicated that chronic use of alcohol stimulated hepatic microsomal enzyme system and increases the metabolism of drugs like warfarin, phenytoin by hepatic microsomal induction. Whereas acute administration of alcohol leads to inhibition of hepatic microsomal enzyme. Concurrent use of alcohol with drugs like sedative, hypnotics, antihistaminics potentiate their effect and leads to excessive depression. Drugs that have interaction with alcohol include cardiovascular agents (isosorbide, nitroglycerine, prazosin, atenolol, verapamil etc.), anxiolytics (alprazolam, diazepam), antidepressants (amytriptyline, imipramine), antidiabetics (metformin, tolbutamide), antibacterials (metronidazole, sulfamethoxazole, fluconazole etc.).

On other hand smoking leads to induction of hepatic microsomal enzyme and leads to excessive metabolic activity of certain category of drugs. Smoking reduces medication effectiveness, makes drug therapy unpredictable and increases risk of side effect. Drugs that have interaction with smoking include cardiovascular agents like beta blockers (propranolol, atenolol etc.), anxiolytic drugs (oxazepam, diazepam), anticoagulants (heparin, warfarin), antiasthmatics (theophylline), antidepressants (imipramine), antipsychotics (haloperidol) etc.

Food and Individual Variation

Food ingested along with drug alters the absorption of drug in various ways. Presence of food affects the rate and extent of drug absorption from gastrointestinal tract. Type of food also has significant importance with respect to absorption of drug. Food containing milk or milk products contains high amount calcium ions which forms complex with drugs like tetracycline and fluoroquinolones. This complex is poorly absorbed in gastrointestinal tract and retards the absorption of these antibiotics. Food material containing substances like tyramine is administered with drugs like MAOI leads to hypertensive reaction. Tyramine is metabolized in intestinal walls by enzyme MAO. Administration of MAOI stops the metabolic degradation of tyramine and significant amount get absorbed in body leading to hypertension.

Even after considering all of the above factors, wide variation is observed in patients towards response to the drug. The reasons behind these variations in response are difficult to explain. Plasma concentration of drugs varies significantly even same group of individual taking same formulation. These variations in response are individual dependent.

Mechanism

Unlike ADR, drug interaction has a definite mechanism of action. Not all the drug interactions listed in text are clinically significant. The individual variation in pharmacokinetics and pharmacodynamic parameters make the patients vulnerable for drug interaction. The degree of drug interaction is also unpredictable and depends on magnitude of drug action. Some patients will be at high risk for drug interaction while other will be less. Geriatric patients are more prone to high risk drug interaction as compared to adult patients. Geriatric patients are more sensitive to the pharmacodynamic effect and their pharmacokinetic parameters are also weak. Moreover geriatric patients required to take more number of drugs as compared to adult due to their multiple disorders, deteriorated health condition.

Pharmaceutical Drug Interactions

Pharmaceutical drug interactions are interactions between two components of formulation before administration of drug formulation to the patient. It is generally represented as incompatibility. Incompatibilities manifest as increase or appearance of haze or turbidity in formulation, development of particulate matter or change in color of formulation. The incompatibility can be physical like physical precipitation or chemical reaction without any change in physical appearance of formulation. There might not be any effect on potency for formulation but majority of time there is loss of potency. The ultimate consequences may leads to very least effect or severe irritation of vein when such formulations are injected. Diazepam injection formulation is prepared using oil based solvent. Dilution of diazepam injection with water for injection or saline leads to precipitation and irritation of tissue when injected as it is. Most of the time in hospitalized patients; drugs were infused with saline solution. Drugs like antibiotics, glucocorticoids, antihistaminics, antiemetics, are infused through saline. These categories of drugs have incompatibility with each other and during infusion all should not be given at once. Each category of drug should be infused one by one. Infusion line must be cleared for first drug and then second drug infusion should be started.

Pharmacokinetic Drug Interactions

Drug interactions that occur at the stage of absorption, distribution, metabolism or excretion are termed as pharmacokinetic drug interactions. Drug interactions of pharmacokinetic type are difficult to detect and are complex in nature. The mechanism behind drug interaction cannot be detected easily. The drug interaction of pharmacokinetic type involves any interaction between drug and other component (drug, food, etc.) leading to change in absorption, distribution, metabolism and/or excretion of drug. The ultimate outcome of pharmacokinetic drug interaction is change in bioavailability (either increased or decreased) of drug at the site of action.

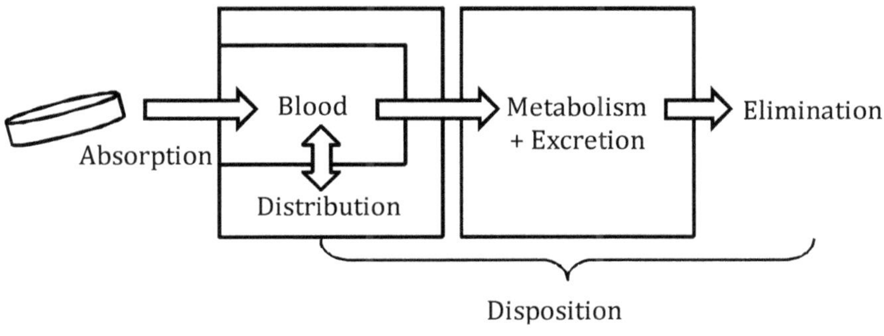

All the pharmacokinetic parameters are divided in to two parts absorption and disposition. Absorption involved entry of drug from site of application to the blood (this excludes direct injection of drug in to blood). Bioavailability is measure of extent of absorption of drug. Disposition comprises of distribution of drug in tissues and its elimination. Elimination itself can be categorized as metabolism and excretion. During direct injection of drug in blood, distribution is independent of absorption. The drug interaction study involves study of mechanism involved in these processes. It involves prediction of quantitative event *in vivo*. Various parameters that contribute in functioning of the above stages involve:

- **Gastric pH:** Most of the drugs are either week acids or week bases. Absorption of drug from gastrointestinal epithelium depends upon the extent to which drug remains in unionized and lipid soluble form. Absorption is hence governed by pKa of drug and its lipid solubility. Acidic drugs are well absorbed in acidic medium because it favors the unionized form and unionized drug get absorbed readily. When drug undergoes in to ionized form (due to change in pH, like acidic drug in alkaline pH or vice versa) its absorption is retarded. The pH of content of gut and various other organs at different levels in gastrointestinal tract is different. This difference in pH differ the absorption of drug in various regions of gastrointestinal tract. Absorption of acidic drug salicylic acid is much greater in acidic pH of stomach as compared to basic pH of intestine.

  Acidic drug ketoconazole requires acidic pH for its dissolution and absorption. Co-administration of antacid or H_2 receptor blockers is likely to reduce the dissolution, absorption and effectiveness of drug as antifungal agent. To avoid this drug interaction it is recommended to administer ketoconazole 2 hr after antacid preparations.

- **Complexation:** Adsorbents are widely used for the treatment of poisoning cases and to remove toxins. Adsorbent invariably reduces the absorption of other drugs also by retarding the absorption of these agents and thereby reduces the therapeutic efficacy of these drugs. Antacids also adsorb some category of drugs and reduced their availability for absorption process. The reduced absorption of the drug molecules by co-administration with antacids or adsorbent is due to complexation, chelation or due to retarded absorption.

Antibiotics like tetracycline, quinolones, penicillamine forms complexation with divalent and trivalent metal ions. Food or drug containing such divalent metal ions forms complex with antibiotic. The metal ion, antibiotic complex is not absorbed through gastrointestinal tract and retards the absorption of antibiotics. The co-administration of tetracycline with food material containing milk and milk products (rich in calcium ions), antacid containing aluminum and magnesium hydroxides, dietary supplements products containing calcium, iron induces this type of drug interaction. The antibiotic - metal ion complex is poorly absorbed. The absorption of tetracycline is retarded and therapeutic efficacy of tetracycline is reduced.

The remedy for such interaction is thought to be discontinuation of one of the drug. But complexation drug interaction can be prevented by administration of drug giving appropriate interval between two administrations. The interval between two administrations should be maximum as possible and minimum of 1 hour elapse. The absorption of doxycycline and minocycline is affected to the lesser extend and compared to tetracycline when co-administered with food containing milk or milk products. However there is significant reduction of absorption of these agents when co-administered with antacid containing aluminum and magnesium hydroxides.

Resinous drugs like cholestyramine, colestipol form complexation with bile acids and retard their absorptions. These two resinous drugs can also form a complex with other drugs present in gastrointestinal tract and hence to reduce the possibility of drug interaction, interval between administrations of these two drugs should be separated as long as possible. Divalent metal ions like aluminum and iron also reduces the absorption of drugs like penicillamine due to complexation. An interval of two hours between their administrations prevents the drug interaction significantly.

- **Gastrointestinal Flora:** Some of drugs when administered undergo inactivation by gastrointestinal bacterial flora. A dose of such drug is decided by considering the fraction which is inactivated in gastrointestinal tract. Co-administration of antibiotics which alters this gastrointestinal microbial flora prevents inactivation of the fraction of drug and leads to more availability and enhanced effect or toxic effect of drug. The phenomenon is more serious when antibiotics are administered with drugs having narrow therapeutic index.

Administration of antibiotic with anticoagulants enhances the effect of anticoagulants and leads to bleeding tendency. Antibiotics interferes with production of vitamin K, poor availability of vitamin K reduces coagulation tendency of blood and normal dose of anticoagulant will leads to poor coagulation of blood and bleeding tendency.

Significant portion of digoxin is converted to parent compound by gastrointestinal microbial flora. This inactivation contributes for reduced activity of digoxin. When antibiotics are administered with digoxin this metabolic conversion is stopped and more fraction of active digoxin is made available for therapeutic effect. The digoxin is drug with very low therapeutic index and hence small variation in blood concentration leads to a toxic effect in patients stabilized on digoxin. On contrary oral contraceptive efficacy is reduced when administered with antibiotics. Oral contraceptives are largely metabolized in liver by conjugation and excreted in bile. The conjugated product is hydrolyzed by intestinal microbial flora and significant amount of free drug is made available and absorbed through intestine. The reduction in microbial flora due to administration of antibiotics prevents hydrolytic cleavage of conjugated oral contraceptive and excreted. This leads to reduction in available oral contractive in systemic circulation.

- **Gastrointestinal motility and gastric emptying:** Absorption of drug depends largely on its residential time of drug in the gastrointestinal tract. If drug stay for large duration of time in gastrointestinal tract its absorption will be significantly enhances. Drugs if move fast in gastrointestinal tract, it does not get enough time for absorption and serum level drops significantly.

  Most of the drugs are absorbed from upper gastrointestinal tract more specifically from stomach. Emptying rate of stomach govern residential time of drug in it and affect the rate of absorption. Altered stomach emptying either enhances or reduces the residential time of drug in stomach and changes its absorption rate. The drugs that alter the stomach emptying rate will have the drug interaction with such drugs and bioavailability will be changes.

Propantheline, reduces the motility of gastrointestinal tract and their by enhances residential time and ultimately bioavailability of drugs like paracetamol, digoxin etc. Paracetamol being a high therapeutic index drug, variation in blood level causes side effects but does not causes life threatening toxic effect. Digoxin has very low therapeutic index and small variation in blood level causes toxicity. On other hand administration of drugs like metoclopramide enhances the motility and retards the rate of absorption of drugs.

A drug which has antimuscarinic effect (as minor therapeutic effect or side effect) reduces gastric motility significantly to cause either enhanced or reduction in rate of absorption of other drug. Tricyclic antidepressants impose antimuscarinic effect on gastrointestinal tract and reduce motility. In presence of tricyclic antidepressants, absorption of dicoumarol is significantly enhanced as time available for dissolution and absorption is significantly increased. On other hand absorption of levodopa is reduced because increased retention of levodopa at gastric mucosa has more time to metabolize the levodopa to dopamine and instead of levodopa, blood level of dopamine rises leading to hypertensive crises.

- **Malabsorption:** Certain drugs like laxatives, cholestyramine causes malabsorption. The state of malabsorption leads to reduced absorption of essential nutrients and vitamins from gastrointestinal tract. This malabsorption state alters the absorption of other drugs if administered simultaneously. Drug like neomycin also produces malabsorption syndrome and impairs the absorption of drugs like digoxin and methotrexate.
- **Presence of food:** Food significantly alters the absorption of drugs from gastrointestinal tract. Absorption of drugs may be delayed but not reduced, but in other case total amount of drug absorbed may be reduced. The delayed absorption of drug in presence of food is due to decreased motility of gastrointestinal tract due to presence of food. Presence of food reduced access of drug to gastric epithelium and reduces rate of absorption. Food also binds the drug and reduces rate of its absorption.

Presence of food also alters the pH of stomach and thereby alters the absorption rate. The presence of food in stomach retards the absorption of drugs like antibiotics, theophyllines, captopril etc., by one or more of the above mechanism.

- **Gastrointestinal metabolism:** Gastrointestinal tract contain microsomal enzymatic system. The rate of absorption of some category of drugs is significantly altered through this microsomal enzymatic system due to metabolism. Serious hypertensive crises have been reported when patients taking tranylcypromine (MAOI) with rich in tyramine containing diet. Tyramine is metabolized by intestinal wall microsomal enzyme MAO and protects us from precursor action of this amine. Administration of MAOI with tyramine rich diet inhibits the enzyme responsible for tyramine metabolism and large amount of amine is accumulated. This excess tyramine releases large quantity of noradrenaline from adrenergic neurons and leads to hypertensive crises.

  Bioavailability of calcium channel blocker (amlodipine), cyclosporine, and HMG-CoA reductase inhibitor (lovastatin) is low due to extensive first pass metabolism. A significant fraction of administered dose from all of these drugs is metabolized by cytochrome P-450 group of enzyme system present in gastrointestinal wall. Consumption of grape fruit juice or other citrus fruit juice significantly elevates the bioavailability of above stated drugs. Grape fruit juice reduces the activity of cytochrome P-450 enzyme system by enzymatic inhibition. This leads to significant reduction in gastrointestinal metabolism of drugs. Due to reduced metabolism, large amount of drug is made available for absorption and contributes for elevated serum concentration of these drug and untoward toxicity.

- **Protein Binding:** The most important cause of drug interaction which involved during distribution is through protein binding. Protein bound drug is displacement of bound drug with another from one or more binding sites. The displacement of one drug by other is competitive process. The amount of drug at the binding site determines the degree of drug displacement. When the molar concentration of a drug at the site of displacement reaches a particular level then only substantial displacement of another drug takes place. The displacement does not depend upon the therapeutic potency of the drug but depends on the amount and affinity of drugs towards protein binding site. Most of the drugs which have capacity to get displaced are potent and hence small displacement also leads to significant alteration in clinical response of drug displaced.

The protein binding might takes place at different sites on protein. The protein binding sites are limited and hence there will be competition for binding at protein binding site. The drug with greater affinity will bind and displaces the drug with other drug from binding site. The protein bound drug is not pharmacologically active and not available for any of the pharmacokinetic or pharmacodynamic phenomenon like distribution, metabolism, excretion, therapeutic effect etc. Plasma protein binding is reversible and equilibrium exists between bound fraction and free fraction of drug. When free drug undergoes metabolism, excretion the equivalent fraction of drug from bound drug will be released in free form.

The risk of drug interaction increases when one victim drug has more plasma protein binding tendency and has a small apparent volume of distribution. In such case very small amount of drug is available as free drug for therapeutic efficacy. Displacement of small percentage of drug from bound fraction will leads to significant alteration of free drug plasma level and hence therapeutic efficacy.

The protein binding and displacement of drug from protein binding site leads to drug interaction. This drug interaction leads to increased or reduced therapeutic effect of victim drug. Phenytoin is significantly displaced from protein site leading to acute elevation of free drug but long term release of this fraction leads to sub therapeutic level and patients suffers epileptic episodes. The free phenytoin fraction of drug is readily metabolized and excreted from body. This rapid metabolism and excretion of drug keep the relative amount of phenytoin in plasma constant and maintain the therapeutic potency, but displaced fraction of drug is lost. This will affect the long term efficacy of drug and at latter stage small amount of drug will be available for equivalent displacement from bound fraction to free drug. The patient will suffer from epileptic episodes after long term exposure to such interaction.

- **Biotransformation:** Very few drugs are excreted from body as it is without metabolism. Most of drugs require metabolic biotransformation before their excretion. Biotransformation takes place by phase one (simple reaction like hydrolysis, reduction, oxidation) and phase two (conjugation with glucuronic acid, sulfonates, glutathione, or amino acids) process. Some drugs require both phase one and phase two metabolism before they could be excreted. This change in drug to its more polar form so as to easy it's excretion are termed as metabolism, biotransformation, biochemical degradation, detoxification etc. Most of the phase one reactions are carried out using cytochrome P-450 enzyme. The metabolic processes are specific for particular category of drug. Some drug shares the common metabolic processes and there will be competition for metabolism at such enzyme site, leading to drug interaction. Some drugs have the tendency to induce or inhibits the metabolic enzyme system and alters the metabolism of victim drug.
- **Enzyme induction:** Many drug interactions are results from enzyme induction of victim drug. The enzyme system necessary for metabolism of drug will be induced and this induced enzymatic system rapidly metabolizes victim drug decreasing the plasma level of drug and sub therapeutic effect.

  Enzyme induction means increased activity of hepatic enzymes, enhanced enzyme synthesis resulting in increased metabolism of victim drug and effective free drug amount. The drugs like barbiturates, rifampin, phenytoin, carbamazepine causes significant enzyme induction.

  Most of the time enzyme induction leads to increased metabolism and detoxification of drug and ultimately reduced therapeutic efficacy of victim drug. There will be rapid reduction in pharmacological action of drug. But by enzyme induction drug might be converted to a more polar and therapeutically more potent drug. This results in potentiation of drug after metabolism. Heavy smoking also leads to enzyme induction of certain category of drug.

- **Enzyme inhibition:** Enzyme inhibition is more common than enzyme induction. In many situations enzyme inhibition results are accumulation, prolongation and intensification of therapeutic effect of victim drug. Unlike enzyme induction, enzyme inhibition occurs early. Enzyme inhibition produces significant outcome within 2 to 3 days and hence results in development of rapid toxicity. Most commonly phase I pathway involving cytochrome P-450 enzyme system is inhibited during process. Phase II conjugation metabolic processes are also inhibited.

  A well known example of metabolic enzyme inhibition that has been useful in clinical practice is use of disulfiram in alcoholism. Disulfiram is inhibitor of enzyme aldehyde dehydrogenase. The enzyme is responsible for oxidative metabolism of alcohol to acetaldehyde. Inhibition of this enzyme by disulfiram leads to accumulation of acetaldehyde. This acetaldehyde develops unpleasant effect, have a typical characteristic disulfiram reaction. Disulfiram also inhibits the enzyme responsible for metabolism of warfarin and phenytoin. Carbamazepine is metabolized by phase II glucuronidation reaction. Sodium valproate inhibits this phase II metabolism and causes toxicity of carbamazepine. Similarly metabolism of azathioprine using phase II methyltransferase reaction is inhibited by aminosalicylates.

- **Biliary excretion and enterohepatic circulation:** Number of drugs were taken up by liver, metabolized for excretion and secreted in bile. The drugs are secreted in bile unchanged or after metabolism as conjugate which make them more polar and water soluble. The drugs having molecular weight more than 450 are excreted largely in the bile. With bile this drug conjugate is secreted in gastrointestinal tract, gastrointestinal microbial flora degrades this conjugates and release free drug which is then again absorbed through intestines in blood circulation. This recycling process of drug is known as enterohepatic circulation and prolongs the stay of drug in blood circulation. Administration of drug that destroys the gastrointestinal microbial flora responsible for degradation of drug conjugate. This leads to excretion of drug conjugate as it is and recycling of drug is stopped.

Hormonal contraceptives are significantly recycles through enterohepatic circulation. Administration of antimicrobials reduces the intestinal microbial flora and stops degradation of drug conjugate leading to early execration of drug and therapeutic efficacy of hormonal contraceptive is reduced.

- **Renal excretion:** Other than inhalation, urinary and biliary excretion is the major site of elimination of most of the drugs. Most of the drugs administered are preferably excreted *via* kidney unchanged or after metabolism. The most important implication during renal excretion takes place when drug is excreted unchanged. The substance is still pharmacologically active and re-absorption of drug contributes for reentry of drug in systemic circulation and ultimately in therapeutic efficacy. In contract, when drug is excreted as inactive metabolite, altered rate of excretion does not affect therapeutic value. Drugs that are bound to plasma proteins are inactive for excretion process.
- **Urinary pH:** Urinary excretion of drug depends on its ionization state. When drug undergo ionization it cannot be reabsorbed. Unionized, lipid soluble drug readily get reabsorbed and reenters in systemic circulation. Urinary pH favors this ionized and unionized state. Acidic drugs remain in unionized form in acidic media while get ionized in basic media. Hence for acidic drug, basic pH favors excretion and acidic pH favors retention in body. Hence the pH at which ionization form of drug is favors, facilitates its excretion.

  Sulfonamide when taken with salts or substances which acidifies the urine leads to chances of development of crystal urea. The excretion of sulfonamides can be facilitated and formation of crystal urea can be prevented by administering of substances that alkalinizes urine.
- **Active urinary transport:** Active transport is the site in renal excretion process where drug is excreted *via* transport pores which are energy dependent and has carrier molecules. Many drugs use same transport system for execration and they compete for excretion process with one another. If such drugs are administered they compete for excretion and affect the excretion of each other.

Penicillin and methotrexate are actively excreted through renal tubules. Administration of probenecid competes with these drugs and prevents their excretion. Instead of penicillin and methotrexate, probenecid itself gets excreted and plasma level of penicillin and methotrexate increases. More over probenecid actively excreted at proximal tubules get reabsorbed at distal end of tubules and hence total outcome is that neither these drugs nor probenecid is excreted and serum concentration of both drugs crosses toxic level.

- **Renal blood flow:** Flow of blood through kidney decides Glomerular Filtration Rate (GFR). This flow of blood through kidney is controlled by vasoconstriction and vasodilatation. Vasodilatation enhances the flow of blood through kidney and thereby GFR. More GFR facilitates the excretion of drug at faster rate hence drugs that increases renal blood flow facilitates excretion of drug while those which reduces blood flow prolongs the drug excretion.

  NSAIDs increase the serum level of lithium leading to toxicity. Prostaglandins are responsible for vasodilation of renal arteries and maintenance of tone. NSAIDs are prostaglandin inhibitors and by this they cause constriction of renal arteries and slowing of renal blood flow. This slowing of renal blood flow reduces the excretion of lithium and serum level of lithium raises leading to toxicity.

Pharmacodynamic Drug Interactions

Pharmacodynamic drug interactions occur most frequently than pharmacokinetic drug interactions. Pharmacodynamic drug interactions are more predictable. These interactions are those where the effect of one drug is altered by other at the site of action. The drug directly competes for the site of action to elucidate therapeutic benefit or the reaction might be more complex involving change in physiological mechanism.

The net outcome of pharmacodynamic drug interaction can be increased overall efficacy also known as synergism or potentiating. The advantage of this type of drug interaction can be taken for clinical benefits. When the overall effect of drug is reduced then the interaction is known as antagonism or inhibition. The advantages of this type of interaction are rare but in some poisoning cases such drug interaction can be beneficial. The third type of outcome of drug interaction is modification or alteration in action. The non expected, unpredictable action will be observed which such drug interaction occurs.

Type	Expression	Example
Additive effect	2 + 2 = 4	Antacid aluminum hydroxide and magnesium hydroxide, Ibuprofen and paracetamol
Synergism	2 + 2 = 6	Trimethoprim and sulphamethoxazole, Levodopa and carbidopa, Isoniazide and rifampicin
Inhibition	2 + 2 = 3	Tetracycline and antacid (containing aluminum, magnesium or calcium salts), Adrenaline and propanolol, Morphine and naloxone
Toxicity	2 + 2 = 9	Digitalis and macrolide antibiotics clarithromycin, Warfarin and aspirin
Modification	2 + 2 = ABC	MAOI (Iproniazid, tranylcypromide) and tyramine rich diet, adrenaline and alpha blockers

- **Additive/Synergism/Potentiation:** Drug interaction when leads to the effect that is equal to mathematical addition of the effect of individual drug when taken alone is termed as additive effect. Drug interaction when leads to more effect than the mathematical addition of the effect of individual drug when taken alone termed as synergism or potentiating action. The synergism leads to enhanced therapeutic effect or toxicity. When therapeutic effect is increases the drug interaction has clinical benefits.

  Alcohol is well known CNS depressant. If taken together with other CNS depressants like sedatives, anxiolytics etc. causes drowsiness. The occurrence of drowsiness is addition of side effect of CNS depressant drugs. The additive effect can occur for both therapeutic effect and/or side effect. When drugs like butyrophenones are given with antipsychotics they share common antimuscarinic action as side effect. Combination of these two drugs precipitates antimuscarinic toxicity.

  The drug combination like trimethoprim and sulphamethoxazole, levodopa and carbidopa, isoniazide and rifampicin are made for getting therapeutic benefits drug interaction. The therapeutic efficacy of combination of these agents is much more than that of efficacy of individual drug. Comparative small amount of drug is required to get therapeutic benefits of individual drug.

- **Opposite/Antagonism/Inhibition:** Antagonism or inhibition type of drug interaction where the combination effect of two drugs is less that the mathematical addition of the effect of individual drug when taken alone. This drug interaction prevents the drug from exerting its action partially or completely and thus diminishes the therapeutic effect of drug on patient. The interaction of drug with opposite effect can be easily detected. Coumarins prolongs the clotting time by inhibiting the vitamin K. Increase in intake of vitamin K counteract the anticoagulant effect of coumarin.
- **Modification:** When the combination of two drugs leads to unexpected results which are beyond the prediction from individual effect of both the drugs leads to modification type of interaction. During synergism or antagonism drug interaction the drug effect is either elevated or reduced. During modification drug interaction the combination effect of two drugs is something other effect than anticipated from two drugs. The combination effect does not have any relation with individual effect of both drugs.

  In Dale's vasomotor reversal phenomenon same drug interaction was found. Adrenaline produces dose dependent elevation of blood pressure. When alpha receptor antagonist is administered before injecting adrenaline the expected effect is that the elevation of blood pressure in lesser degree. But unexpectedly severe fall in blood pressure is observed. In therapeutics when given individually neither adrenaline nor alpha receptor blockers produces fall in blood pressure. The fall in blood pressure is due to blocked of alpha receptor and exposure of selective beta receptors (as adrenaline is non selective adrenergic agonist) leading to fall in blood pressure.

Drug Interaction Studies

Drug interaction should be considered and studied from the perspective of both newly developed drug and new drug under development (investigational drug) and drug which is already been used in the clinical practice. It is always possible that new drug will interact with established drug. Drug interaction should be viewed from perspective of both the drugs. Any one or both of the drugs can be affected due to such interactions. When drug has to be used as a component of combination or prescribed with other drug formulation then the possibility of occurrence of drug interaction, effect of such interaction on clinical efficacy should thoroughly assessed. Based on the results of pharmacokinetic, toxicity and pharmacological studies, clinical and non-clinical interaction studies should be conducted for examining drug interaction.

When the concentration of drug in plasma is very low and below detectable limit then possibility of presence of major metabolite should be checked for evaluation of drug concentration in plasma. The undetected amount of drug or metabolite might be sufficient to cause the major drug interaction. The physicochemical property, pharmacological actions, pharmacokinetic behavior and clinical usage of each drug differ for other drug. The method and protocol for drug interaction study for such drugs should be selected appropriately depending on the property of drug under investigational consideration.

From the pharmacokinetic perspectives the factors that are responsible for drug interactions should be taken in to consideration prior to conduct of clinical studies. The clinical study protocol should be designed in such a way that all the possible information of drug interaction as a consequence of co-administration of both drugs should be obtained. It is also important to consider the clinical dose, route of administration of both the drugs during such studies. These clinical studies should be conducted as per strict guidelines of good clinical practice and other guidelines given by appropriate authorities.

Drug - Food Interaction

Many time it is a wrong notion that drug do not interact with food. Food materials are neutral in interaction with drugs. But it is not true. Very often food and drug interaction lead to unwanted circumstances. Hence it is always suggested that while taking the drugs, interaction of drug with food should be taken in to account. The medication taken by mouth travels same path where food is passing and there is possible chance that during their passage they will interact with each other. It will be mistaken to consider the vitamins, dietary supplements or herbal formulation as food components. Drug – food interaction takes place when ingredients of drug interact with food material. The drug – food interaction become high risk, when such interaction takes place in geriatric patients. The chances of drug – food interaction are always more in geriatric patients because they take more number of medicines as compared to adults due to their multiple abnormal conditions like diabetes, hypertension, high cholesterol, congestive heart diseases etc. In such condition patients monitoring is very essential for drug – food interactions.

The drug – food interaction has gain importance in health care system. Certain food stuffs alter the absorption, bioavailability, pharmacokinetics and pharmacodynamics and therapeutics of medications. Moreover therapeutic efficacy of some drugs depends on nutritional status of the patients. In sum, presence or absence of food in gastrointestinal tract affect the drug action due to drug – food interaction. Drug – food interaction can happen with both prescription and non prescription drugs. Any component present in drug that has capability to interact with any component of food leads to unexpected outcomes.

Like food material drug is also absorbed through the epithelial linings of the gastrointestinal tract. Mostly presence of food in gastrointestinal tract retards absorption of drug. Hence drug must be taken in empty stomach for better absorption. However drug which produces irritation needs presence of food otherwise may cause adverse complications like hyperacidity or gastric ulceration. Presence of dietary fibers retards the absorption of drug. For example, injection of pectin containing food with pain killer paracetamol slows the absorption of drug. Food containing large amount of vitamin K, promotes formation of blood clot and counteract the effect of anticoagulants like heparin.

Dietary supplements contain excess of vitamins, minerals, amino acids and essential inorganic components. Any of these components can interact with prescription or non prescription drug leading to drug – food interaction. Consumption food material like coffee, chocolate containing xanthenes if taken with drugs like theophylline in treatment of asthma leads to increased toxicity of theophylline. Alcohol containing beverages interacts with antidepressants and other CNS depressing agents and affects brain function.

Clinical Perspective

In last 1 to 20 years discovery of drugs in the area of selective serotonin reuptake inhibitor, mixed mechanism antidepressants, azole antifungal agents, newer macrolide antibiotics, high reactive antiretroviral agents, drugs acting on human immunodeficiency virus introduced many molecules in the clinical practice. These molecules have a complex pharmacokinetic and pharmacodynamic behavior in human body. Due to this complex nature of these drugs considerable attention has been paid towards interaction of these drug molecules with other drug molecules and food components. These categories of drugs have major impact on clinical practice as life saving drug while complex nature of these drugs have increased the chance of occurrence of drug interaction. These drugs have secondary pharmacological effects like enzyme induction or inhibition which also contributes for drug interactions.

One of the objectives of drug development study is to generate data which will help physician to assist the clinical use of drug. The objective of generation of information related to drug interaction for its possible safe use is overlooked most of the time. More attention is paid on therapeutic efficacy of these drugs. Because the possible numbers of interaction are very large and time and resources available to generate this information (pharmacokinetic and pharmacodynamic drug interactions) is limited, the generated drug interaction data might be inappropriate. The drug interaction studies are either postponed till phase IV of clinical trials or might be bypassed in total.

In technical/scientific language the drug that cause drug interaction is called as "perpetrator" while the drug which is being affected in called as "victim". In the pharmacokinetic drug interaction perpetrators alter metabolism or clearance of victim in systemic circulation leading to elevated or decrease concentration of drug in body. Pharmacokinetic drug interactions are one where the perpetrator is not changed at all. In pharmacodynamic interactions, victim drug is inhibited or Induced for its clinical efficacy.

Human cytochrome P450 (CYP) is group of enzyme responsible for major metabolic activities. Different mechanisms are involved in induction and inhibition of these enzymes. Enzyme inhibition involved direct chemical effect on CYP enzyme, rapid onset of inhibition, reversible inhibition and immediate exposure of enzyme with drug is needed and prior exposure of enzyme with drug is not needed. In enzyme inhibition process mechanism involved is indirect and through enhanced quantity of CYP protein, onset of induction is slow, inhibition is practically irreversible, immediate exposure is not needed and prior exposure of drug is must. A drug that induces and inhibits the CYP might influence both hepatic and gastrointestinal CYP not in same degree. Unique example of drug is ritonavir which act as both inducer as well as inhibitor. The drug enzyme reaction (inducer/inhibitor) is time dependent. Initial exposure of ritonavir with CYP leads to inhibition, while exposure for prolonged duration of time is counterbalanced by enzyme induction. The net outcome is initial inhibition and after prolonged period of time unpredictable no effect or induction of enzyme system.

During clinical practice multiple administration of more than one drug is most common. Non interaction of these co-administered drug is more common than interaction. During such non interaction also some degree of pharmacokinetic and/or pharmacodynamic interaction takes place but have no clinical significance. When these interactions aggravate due to some reason the drug interaction in precipitated and clinical intervention becomes must.

Toxicological Perspective

Unanticipated drug action in the clinical practice by the drug after their introduction in to market due to its clinical use in large degree of population is a major problem. The new drug produces immunological reactions leading to toxicity. The new drug might be perpetrator or victim. The narrow therapeutic index of the drug makes it a potential candidate for drug interaction. In such case small variation in the systemic concentration leads to large change in pharmacokinetic or pharmacodynamic profile of drug and leads to drug interactions. The narrow therapeutic index of a drug means a drug which has less than two fold difference between median lethal dose and median effective dose.

Majority of drug interaction occurs by interaction with CYP level. Available information revel that induction or inhibition of these enzyme system is potential cause of these drug interactions. Many metabolic drug interactions can be predicted during clinical trials of the drug through systematic study of alteration in metabolic status. However factors like genetic and individual variation, environmental factors, physiological variations, nature of diet had a major influence on occurrence of toxicological consequences of drug interaction.

Anticoagulant drug like warfarin have narrow therapeutic index, and extensive metabolic oxidative inactivation using enzyme system CYP. Hence warfarin is most prone for drug interaction by enzyme induction or inhibition. Enzyme inducer drugs like barbiturates, phenytoin increases the demand of high dose to achieve same therapeutic effect, on other hand drugs like sulphonamide, metronidazole, some antifungal agents act as enzyme inhibitor and leads to life-threatening bleeding consequences. The requirement of drug is reduced due to enzyme inhibition and patients take normal dose leading to increased level of drug in systemic circulation and excessive therapeutic effect. Clinically enzyme induction and inhibition become important when patient is stabilized on a specific dose of warfarin. This alteration in enzyme *via* induction or inhibition either elevates or decreases the required therapeutic level of anticoagulant and leads to clinical complications.

Benzodiazepines are widely used as sedative, hypnotics and anxiolytics in clinical practice and extensively used by CYP3A enzyme system. Co-administration of drugs which induces or inhibits these enzyme system leads to marked alteration in plasma concentration and leads to toxic effect such as deep sleep, unconsciousness etc. or precipitates the symptoms of diseases.

Cardio-tonic digitalis has narrow therapeutic index. A significant fraction of digitalis gets metabolized during its absorption through gastrointestinal tract. Administration of antibiotics which kills the intestinal microbial flora reduces this metabolism and more digitalis is available for systemic absorption. This elevated level of digitalis contributes for toxicity.

Drug having narrow therapeutic index causes serious toxic effects, when undergo drug interaction. The drug interactions cause significant alteration in tissue drug concentration and causes toxicity and hence limit their usefulness. Most of these drug interactions occur at metabolic level. It is still unclear whether the metabolic status or immunological reactions of drug due to elevated concentration is responsible for toxicological consequences after drug interaction.

Metabolic Enzymes and Drug Interactions

Cytochrome P450 contributes for phase 1 metabolic process. This group of enzyme is present primarily in liver and small intestine. In minor quantity it is also present in lungs, kidney, brain and heart. Majority of drugs were eliminated unchanged *via* various routes like renal, gastrointestinal or pulmonary. The fraction excreted unchanged is around 25%. CYP mediated metabolism includes 55% fraction, and other metabolism by other process includes 20%. CYP are omnipresent in nature. They are found in bacteria, plant, mammals and more than hundred types of CYP are invented. They show species or even tissue specific function. Human Cytochrome P450 subfamily is based on number of enzymes, substrates attached to each enzyme. Each subtype of enzyme show 40% homology in sequence of amino acids are place in one same family and if homology is more than 60% then enzyme is placed in same subfamily.

CYP is found throughout body, particularly at interface such as intestine, epithelium, skin etc. liver and intestinal epithelium is predominant site where CYP are found. CYP is also found where drug is eliminated. Hence consideration of CYP and its activity is worth during drug interaction study. Many different types of CYP are found in intestine. Multiple factors such as smoking, alcoholism, environmental factors, disease state and genetic inheritance influence the amount and activity of CYP in human body. CYP play a major role in metabolism and elimination of many drugs. Many drugs like cyclosporine, midazolam, felodipine were metabolized by CYP3A4. Grapefruit juice has potential effect on enzyme CP3A4 and alters the metabolism and elimination of these drugs leading to a potential drug interaction. The CYP group of enzyme is inducible by environmental factors such as cigarette smoking. CYP enzymes also metabolize several drug substrates. The patients with liver cirrhosis have decreased drug metabolizing capacity due to reduced amount of CYP. The degree to which amount of CYP are reduced is not uniform. The down regulation of CYP is also observed during inflammation and infection leading to patients becomes more susceptible for drug interactions.

CYP group of enzyme is responsible for microsomal drug metabolism, biosynthesis, degradation of drug molecules, endogenous compounds. The CYP performs verity of chemical reactions including oxidation, reduction, hydrolysis, conjugation etc. to make them more water soluble so as to facilitate their elimination from the body. The prodrug activation is also done by CYP biotransformation process. In phase 1 metabolic processes addition of simple groups like hydroxyl, amine or sulfhydryl is done using CYP. The product of phase 1 metabolism may undergo excretion or participate in phase 2 metabolic process where conjugation reaction takes place. In conjugation reaction the drug or substrate is conjugated with large substrate molecules like glucuronic acid, glutathione, sulfur or glycine. The product of phase 2 metabolic process is highly polar and excreted in urine readily. This same pathway is also followed for the metabolism of endogenious biological substances like hormones, cholesterol, eicosanoids, bile salts and bile acids. Thus there will be competition for the metabolic process between drug and biological substance. Drug interaction leads to hampering of metabolism of either drug molecule or biological substances.

Role of Pharmacist

Large numbers of drugs are introduced in clinical therapy every year. Drug interaction has received a great deal of attention for regulatory, scientific, health care community. It is impossible for physician to memorize all aspects of these drugs during clinical practice. The consequences of drug interaction lead to death, life-threatening effect, hospitalization, disability (temporary or permanent) and hence require intervention to prevent them. Depending on the consequences the drug interactions can be termed as sever, serious.

All health care professional (especially pharmacist) has a prime duty to ensure that patient will get safe medicine, and they should be aware of the unwanted consequences of it. A due care and measures must be taken when such unwanted consequences (like drug interaction) were observed or reported. Pharmacists have detailed knowledge about medicine, and have ability to correlate the unexpected consequences observed or reported by the patients during drug therapy. The pharmacist has to play a major role in detection, reporting and prevention of such drug interactions.

Drug interactions between some classes of drugs are well-known. Pharmacist should suggest suitable alternative if prescribing such drugs is must during clinical practice. Some time it is possible to give two interacting drugs by adjusting the dose or administration frequency or timing. Interacting drugs can also administered by keeping sufficient time interval between administrations of two drugs. In some cases close monitoring of the patients clinically and with the help of laboratory data will also help in administering the interacting drugs. The appropriate change in dose or substituting the one of the drug will help to avoid drug interaction. Pharmacist has the knowledge of this and such interacting drugs can be given with consultation of pharmacist. Pharmacodynamic drug interactions can be anticipated based on knowledge of clinical effect of drugs. Pharmacokinetic drug interactions are difficult to anticipate. They cannot be predicted from their pharmacological or clinical effect. The drug interactions were based more on physicochemical properties of the drug molecule.

It has been found by clinician and pharmacist that patients do not report the occurrence of consequences of drug interactions even though observed. Patient thinks that it is the integral part of therapy. Such consequences of drug interactions can be avoided by the pharmacist through counseling the patients during follow up visits. The computerization of drug interaction data and patients prescription record can help the pharmacist in guiding and avoiding such drug interactions.

The database or computerized drug information about drug interaction contains possible interaction between two drugs when administered to the patients. The consequence of drug interaction is not only depends on the interaction between two drugs but also other factors beyond the scope of reaction between two drugs. Several factors other than two drugs contributes for occurrence and severity of drug interactions are patients related and includes age, physiology, genetics, lifestyle, diet, exercise, underlying disease, alcoholism or smoking etc. For the effective control on prevention of drug interaction pharmacist should take some preventive measures which includes:

- Preparation of medication plan and its implementation, which include selection of medicament, modification in medicament if needs?
- Monitoring and evaluating the response of patients to therapeutic regimen (therapeutic drug monitoring).

- Identification, compiling, resolving and preventing medication related problems by performing comprehensive review which includes adverse drug events.
- Delivering, communicating and documenting the relevant essential information to the patients and other health care professionals.
- Providing verbal information and training for patients understanding.
- Providing information, support service, resources for enhancement of patient's adherence.
- Provide the complete information about the medication, diet and other supplements taken by the patient to the health care professional.
- To provide health care professional information about commencement, termination, modification (if any) in the medication, change in lifestyle (diet, exercise, starting/discontinue of alcohol/smoking).

References

Adrian Belîi, Natalia Belîi (2010). Drug interactions in anaesthesia practice: a basic review for residents. *Anestezjologia* **4:** 99-110.

Ansari J.A. (2010). Drug Interaction and pharmacist. *Journal of Young Pharmacists* **2(3):** 326-331.

Avoid food-drug interaction, A guide from National consumers league and U.S. Food and Drug Administration, (website: www.nclnet.org or www.fda.gov/drugs).

Baravkar A.A, Sawant S.D, Bhise S.B, Dhabale P.N (2009). Herb-Drug Interactions. *Indian J. Pharm. Pract.* **2(2):** 25-30.

Ben D Snyder, Thomas M Polasek, Matthew P Doogue (2012). Drug interactions: principles and practice. *Australian Prescriber* **35:** 85-88.

Chris Raich, Drug Interactions, West Virginia University Extension Service, WLG 410.

Chrischilles E.A, Fulda T.R, Byrns P.J, Winckler S.C, Rupp M.T, Chui M.A (2002). The role of pharmacy computer systems in preventing medication errors. *J Am Pharm Assoc* **42:** 439-448.

Daniel E. Becker (2011). Adverse Drug Interactions. *Anesth Prog* **58:** 31-41.

David J Woods, New Zealand College of Pharmacists, Introduction to Drug Interactions.

Doucet J, Chassagne P, Trivalle C, Landrin I, Pauty MD, Kadri N (1996). Drug-drug interactions related to hospital admissions in older adults: A prospective study of 1000 patients. *J Am Geriatr Soc.* **44:** 944-948.

Drug and the therapeutic science (Drug-Drug interactions) edited by A. David Rodrigues, Vol. 116, Marcel Dekker, Inc, New York.

Guideline for industry, Drug Interaction studies – study design, data analysis, implications for dosing, and labeling recommendations, U.S. Department of Health and Human Services, Food and Drug Administration, Centre for Drug Evaluation and Research (CDER), (Feb. 2012). Clinical Pharmacology (website: http://www.fda.gov/Drugs/GuidanceComplianceRegulatoryInformation/Guidances/default.htm).

Hazlet TK, Lee TA, Hansten PD, Horn JR (2001). Performance of community pharmacy drug interaction software. *J Am Pharm Assoc* **41:** 200-204.

Henry J. Mann (2006). Drug-Associated Disease: Cytochrome P450 Interactions. *Crit Care Clin* **22:** 329-345.

J. L. Bauman (2001). The role of pharmacokinetics, drug interactions and pharmacogenetics in the acquired long QT syndrome. *European Heart Journal Supplements* 3(Supplement K) K93-K100.

Jaclyn Thu-Nguyet Nguyen (2004). Pharmacist: practitioner or provider?

L. Magro & A. Conforti & F. Del Zotti & R. Leone & M. L. Iorio & I. Meneghelli & D. Massignani & E. Visonà & U. Moretti (2007). Identification of severe potential drug-drug interactions using an Italian general-practitioner database. *Eur J Clin Pharmacol* 7.

Louise Mallet, Anne Spinewine, Allen Huang (2007). Prescribing In Elderly People 2, The challenge of managing drug interactions in elderly People. *Lancet* **370:** 185-91.

Marta Sousa, Anton Pozniak and Marta Boffito (2008). Pharmacokinetics and pharmacodynamics of drug interactions involving rifampicin, rifabutin and antimalarial drugs. *Journal of Antimicrobial Chemotherapy* **62:** 872-878.

Methods of drug interaction studies. A official text document in Japanese intended for use as a reference in conducting drug interaction studies.

Mohammad Yaheya Mohammad Ismail (2009). Drug-Food Interactions and Role of Pharmacist. *Asian Journal of Pharmaceutical and Clinical Research* **2(4)**.

Ogbru O (1996). Drug-food interactions. *Clin Trends Pharm Pract* **10:** 53-60.

Ogbru O (1997). Drug interactions with grapefruit juice. *Drug Links* **1:** 59-60.

Orloff DG (2002). Label changes for Simvastatin (Zocor) US Food and Drug Administration.

Philip N. Patsalos, Walter Froscher, Francesco Pisani, Clementina M. van Rijn (2002). The Importance of Drug Interaction in Epilepsy Therpay. *Epilepsia* **43(4):** 365-385.

Remington (2005). The Science & Practice of Pharmacy, 21st ed, Lippincott Williams & Wilkins.

Singh Arjun, Sharma Raju, Anand Kunwar Manu, Khan Shaheen Praveen and Sachan Naresh Kumar (2012). Food-drug interaction. *International Journal of Pharmaceutical and chemical science* **1(1):** 264-269.

Singh Nishi, Concept of drug Interaction (2012). *International Research Journal of Pharmacy* **3(7)**.

Stockley (2008). Drug Interactions, edited by Karen Baxter, 8th ed, PhP Pharmaceutical Press.

CHAPTER 7

Patients Counseling

Introduction

A patient takes the medicine for cure, diagnosis and mitigation of illness. The goal of safe and effective use of drug can only be active, if the patients are well aware about the medicine, their use and other effect if not taken appropriately. Knowledge of patient about medicine improves compliance for effective utilization of drug. The improved compliance improves therapeutic outcomes. Pharmacist is well aware about drugs that patient should know and hence pharmacist plays important role for patient's education regarding medicine. Most of the time due to illness patient is not in mental status of listening to anyone and in such condition patients counseling by pharmacist plays a vital role. Pharmacist must be fully aware about his role in patients counseling. Pharmacist should counsel the patient for education regarding medicine that will help patient to have safe and effective therapy. It will help patients for avoiding intentional and unintentional misuse of medicine and improves the compliance. This all can be achieved effectively through patients counseling.

Counseling means giving advice, consultation, opinion, suggestion and knowledge to the patient about medicine and illness. Patients counseling is a process of sympathetic interaction between patient/ customer/consumer and health care professionals, especially pharmacist. Initially counseling was done by priests in churches. At later stage leader of society take this responsibility as a social obligation. Now a day it is done in hospitals and pharmacy. Patient counseling helps for effective and safe use of medicine, understanding drug interactions, instruction giving for medicine administration, follow-up etc. Patients counseling become more important during multiple drug therapy. Pharmacist can also advice patient regarding financial aspect related to drug therapy, reimbursement, insurance schemes, health benefit policy etc.

Function and Scope

Patients counseling involves transmitting information regarding medicine to the patient when patient do not want to intend it due to any reason. The counseling contains information and advice that should be properly understood by patient. The information and advice should be transmitted in the language and words which must be understood by the patient. A suitable media must be selected for counseling of the patient. The media selection depends of the patient. Audiovisual films, projectors, interactive boards can be used effectively in the patients who are friendly with audiovisual aids, computer systems. Illiterate patients and patients who are not friendly with electronic gazettes may not be friendly with utilization of these systems. In such cases verbal communication and non interactive films may be helpful and give effective outcome. The component involved in patients counseling are shown in figure below.

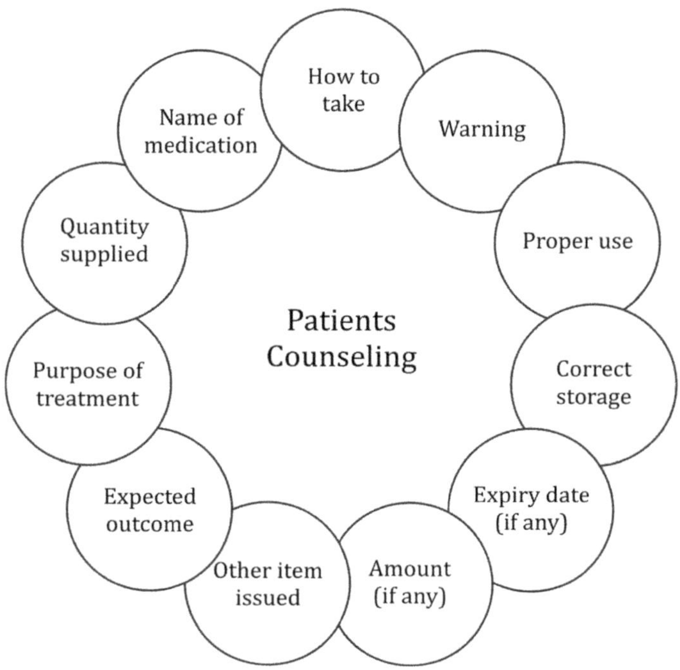

The pharmacist counsels the patient, representative or guardian about following during drug regimen.

- Name and identification of medicine, trade name, generic name etc.
- Way by which the medicine should be taken. Route of administration, frequency, time and schedule of administration etc.
- Special precautions to be taken during drug administration like: to be taken before or after meal, avoiding milk and milk product etc. Expected side effect, idea about drug interaction etc.
- Special instruction for appropriate use of medicine. For example, tablet to be chewed, swallowed or kept under tongue.
- Appropriate storage condition of medication like keep in cool and dry place, keep in refrigerator etc.
- Expiry date of medicine. For example, reconstituted suspension must be used within one month after opening container. Sterile ophthalmic preparations should be used within one month after opening the container.
- The information regarding cost of drug, reimbursement, cost effective alternates etc.
- Along with container of dosage form some time other accessories/items are also supplied. Appropriate use of such items must be explained. Measuring containers as cap of bottle, application for gel or creams etc.
- The therapeutic drug requires some time to cure disease. It will take certain time for this. Outcome will be visualized after specific period of time and depends of type of illness and medicine prescribed. The information regarding expected out come and time required for it should be clearly informed to patient.
- The purpose of treatment, aim and objective behind prescribing each medicine.
- The quantity of medicine supplied, re-filling information. The quantity and frequency of administration determine the duration of treatment.
- All other information found relevant, appropriate and necessary for effective use of therapy.

Patients counseling provides benefits to patients as well as to the pharmacist. The patient will understand medicine in better scene and have better understanding of his medicine which will benefit him during pharmacotherapy. This will have following benefits.

- Better therapeutic outcomes and minimal adverse drug indications.
- Better patient's adherence during pharmacotherapy.
- Reduced misuse and errors in medication.
- Involvement of patient in therapy, improves self management and help in early recovery.
- Appropriate use of medicine reduces cost of treatment.

The benefits to the pharmacist includes

- Enhanced professional status in the view of patient and other health care professionals.
- Establishment of himself as an important component of health care provider team. The position cannot be replaced by any other professionals.
- Improved patients outcome gives enhanced job satisfaction.
- Can give value added services to the patients and become an important member of health care team.
- Improved revenue generation through patients counseling. Presently this factor does contribute negligible in Indian context but it is growing very fast.

As per the US medication Counseling Behavior Guidelines, after a patient counseling it is expected that following desirable outcome must be obtained.

- Patient should recognize why medicine is prescribed for him. How the prescribed medicine is going to help in cure and mitigation of illness.
- Patient will accept relationship between health care professional team members and cooperate with and support to team member during therapy. This improved relation become basis for continued interaction and consultation.
- Improves patient's adherence to medication by better understanding the medication related decisions.

- Increased strength to deal with medicine related adverse drug reactions and drug interactions.
- Patient's active participation in treatment of illness and self care will be improved due to increased information and efficiency.
- Improved health status shows motivation of patient.

Factors that should be taken into account during counseling process includes age of patient, language which the patient understands, medication history of patient and category of medicine prescribed for patient.

- **Age:** Geriatric patients have forgetful nature and require assistance. Also they have to take several medicines simultaneously for multiple age related disorders.
- **Language:** Patients who are illiterate, does not have knowledge about English requires additional counseling.
- **Medication history:** Patients prescribed with medicine should be asked about his previous by prescribed, OTC medicine. Patient might take medicine for so long period of time that he forgets to tell about that medicine.
- **Category of medicine:** Certain category of drugs requires counseling. When patient is taking supplementary medicine, herbal products or dietary supplement products requires counseling to avoid any interaction. Medicine with common side effect requires counseling to minimize them. Medicine when requires complex procedures for administration, special storage precautions, when therapeutic index is low the counseling is must.

Skills and Techniques

For effective patients counseling some skills and techniques has to be applied. Following are some skills and techniques used for effective patients counseling.

- **Communication skill:** Information can be communicated from sender to receiver by various ways. Verbal and non-verbal communications are two principle modes of the communication process. Use of verbal communication includes use of language, tone, volume, pitch and speed of speech. Language chosen for communication should be such that patient should easily understood. The use of friendly language for patient helps him in better way for understanding. Depending on situation tone of speaking should be varied. Geriatric patients might have hearing problem and use of high tone is required. Ideally counseling should be done in quiet and private environment. Clarity and understanding of speech depends on rate of speed of communication. High speed speaking might give impression that pharmacist is too busy and he does not have enough time for counseling. On other hand if pharmacist speaks too slowly, the patient may lose interest in communication.

Other than verbal communication process pharmacist and patients communicate *via* non-verbal way of communication. Eye contact, facial expressions, facial features are factors that contributes in effective communication process. Blank start, nervousness, inattentiveness, interruptions, disturbance are barriers of effective communication. Touch, although a part of non verbal communication enhances the verbal communication process. Greeting with handshake by pharmacist is a part of introduction but touch attends the patients comfort. Touch displays sympathy, empathy, concern and attention. Holding the hand of pediatric or geriatric patient during communication gives them confidence for effective communication. Pharmacist should use his skill, experience and knowledge for effective communication during patients counseling.

- **Listening skill:** Listening to the patients is hard but extremely important during patient's counseling. Pharmacist should allow patient to speak freely and without interruption. Pharmacist should encourage patients who hesitate to speak about their illness. Pharmacist should concentrate on wards, meaning of what patients want to speak. Pharmacist should avoid direct jumping on the conclusion from discussion. Proper listening from patient will give idea about various aspect of illness of patient even if it is not communicated verbally.

- **Questioning skill:** Questioning skill of pharmacist can be used for extracting the desired information from the patient. Open ended question should be asked where patient cannot give the answer yes or no. Patient has to think and explain in detail for answering the question. Open ended questions starts with who, what, where, when, why, how etc. When precise answer is required leading question or restricting questions were asked. The answers were predetermined rather than explanatory from patient. Questions usually supplied with hints about answer to the patients.
- **Paraphrasing:** Paraphrasing is reforming the sentence of patient by pharmacist in his own words and language. This gives idea to the patient that pharmacist has listened and understood what he has held him and the message was received by pharmacist accurately. Paraphrasing listening is also known as active listening. Paraphrasing listening allows the patients to check that pharmacist have listen him correctly or not. This is one way pharmacist can build the confidence and relation between pharmacist and patient's effective communication.
- **Technical language:** During the process of patients counseling special techniques must be used by pharmacist to make the patient understand. Unnecessary use of technical terms and language can create anxiety in the patient. When use of technical term is mandatory the meaning of it should be explain separately. Pharmacist commonly use language full of medical terminology, Latin wards, names of medicines, abbreviations, Greek prefix. This language can easily understand by other health care professionals but creates great confusion and anxiety in patients. During communicating with patients, pharmacist must keep this limit in mind. Pharmacist should use appropriate common language word instead of specific term. When it becomes impossible to substitute or mandatory to use such word then the meaning of such word should be explain to the patient separately.
- **Organization of sessions:** The session of patients counseling should be designed in logical manner and it aim at extracting

the desired information from patients. The sequence and logic of questioning should be designed scientifically. The flow of information should logical from one issue to the next. The sequence of question should be structured such that it should flow from simple conceptual to logical and complex. Use of standard format is also advisable in many circumstances. It will help pharmacist to develop technique and standard protocol for patents counseling. Disorganized questioner increases the chances of repeating question or increased chance of likelihood questions. This might also miss some important questions and appropriate information may not be obtained from patient. In replying such question patient might become confused if questioner jump around same issue for longer period of time.

- **Control of session:** For successful patients counseling sufficient information must be gathered. To gather necessary information sufficient time must be permitted during counseling. Pharmacist must direct the session effectively towards the main topic when patient is far away from the purpose of the session.
- **Use of written information:** For effective retention of information use of multiple modes of communication is most effective. Verbal communications are easy to understand but memorization power of listeners affects its outcome. Pharmacist can supply ancillary label on the main container of medicine, where he can put additional information about the schedule of drug and dose administration. Use of fluorescent highlighter can grasp the attention on critical point of information.

Counseling Process

The process of counseling starts with listening and understanding the doubt of the patient. This must involves sympathetic listening and understanding of doubts, problems and views of patient regarding illness. These doubts, problems and views must be understood in professional manner. The interaction with patient during counseling process should be sympathetically. The counseling should be done in adequate privacy. Area used for counseling should be semi-private, with special, comfortable sitting arrangement. The counseling talk must be initiated by pharmacist with introduction. Listening to the patient should be paraphrasing, encouraging to the patient. Pharmacist should clarify doubt and listen to the patient enthusiastically. Non-verbal communication should include eye contact, nodding head etc. Counselor must be listener, education provider, facilitator, and acceptor. He should not argue, should not behave like a judge and should not talk or make statement which will adversely affect the therapeutics. Multiple questioning, irrelevant questions, judgment attitude, showing importance should be avoided during counseling. The logical sequence of patient counseling is given in the figure below.

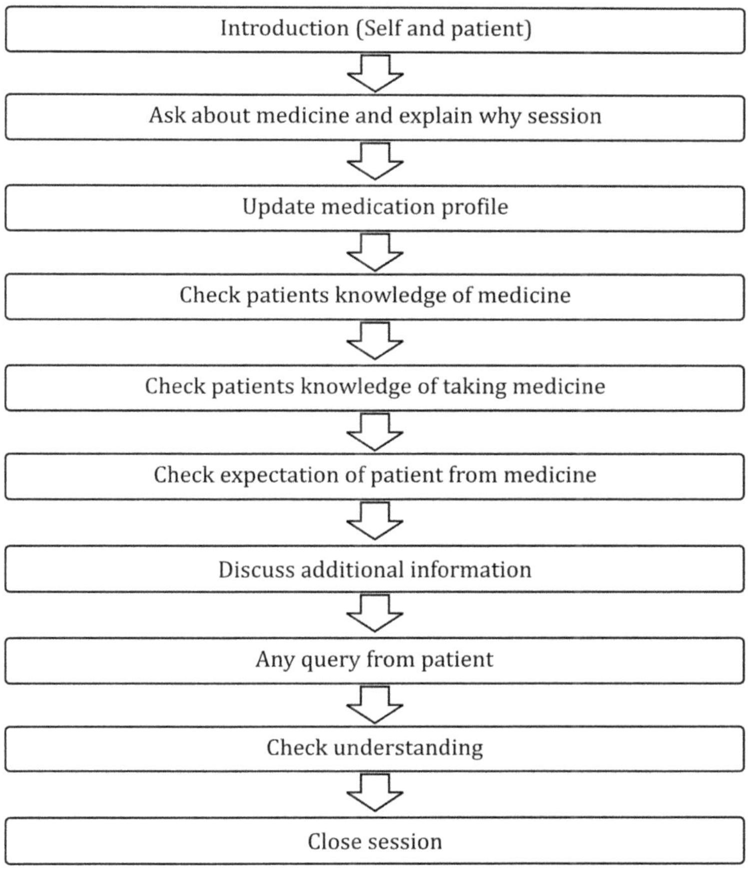

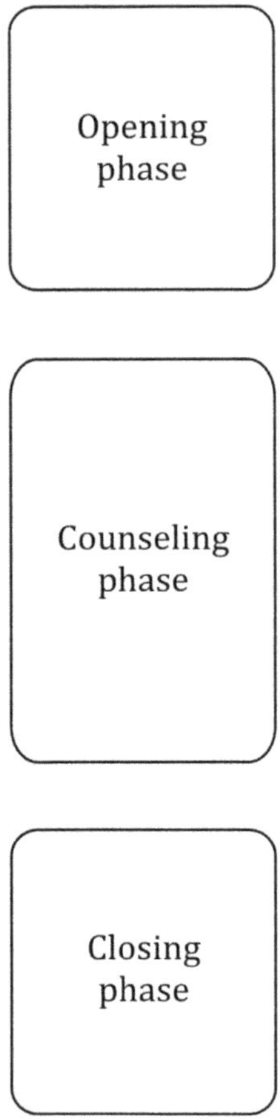

The process of counseling takes place in three phases and comprises of around 10 steps. The first 3 steps of phase 1 includes introduction with patient, asking patient about medicine and updating patients medication record. In phase 1 no communication takes place in order to counsel the patient. Phase 2 is actually a counseling phase which takes place step by step. It begins with checking patient's knowledge about medicine and administration of medicine. The process continued with understanding and fulfilling the expectation of patient regarding information of medicine. The next step in counseling involves additional information that patient requires or must know about medicine. The phase of counseling ends here and phase 3 consist of closing of counseling. Steps involved in phase 3 include asking queries if any from patient, checking whether patient understood the communication or not and closing of session as well as counseling process.

1. **Introduction:** Communication for effective counseling should start with introduction by pharmacist himself. Greet the patient with smile on face and offer hand in appreciation. Provide your name with position. Identify the person to whom you should speak. It is best practice to put title before patients name like Mr. Mrs. Miss. etc. with first name of patient. For example. "Hello Mr. Avinash! I am Mukesh, your pharmacist. I would like to tell you about medicine, which doctors have prescribed to you".
2. **Ask about medicine and explain why medicine:** In this stage pharmacist gather information about patients understanding regarding illness and medicine prescribed for him. Pharmacist should ask few simple questions to know the fact regarding whether patient know about illness, medicine intend to take, any other OTC medicine he is taking etc. Explain the patient about purpose, importance of treatment. Patient if do not receive counseling properly may make mistake taking medicine and treatment may not go effectively. Counseling of such patients enhances the chances of patient adherence to the medicine. Pharmacist should also extract the information regarding allergic condition, contraindication for certain category of medicine and history of medicine taken in previous etc.
3. **Update medication profile:** Upon receiving all this information, pharmacist should update all the information or any change in previously recorded information in database or it should be kept in written format on paper for updating in later stage. This collection must include information about allergy, disease state, new and discontinued prescription medicines and non-prescription medicines, dietary supplements, herbal products, history about change in social/lifestyle.
4. **Check patients knowledge of medicine:** The actual process of counseling starts from this stage. If patients want to know, it is the legal right to know about the medicine prescribed for him. Pharmacist should ask the patient why he was in clinic and why prescription was given to him. Simple questions will give idea about nature of illness and knowledge of patient regarding the medicine intended for him. See that patient know the purpose of medication, correct name of medicine prescribed and strength. This is the time pharmacist should introduce patient with

prescribed medicine. Pharmacist should physically show the bottle/strip of medicine to the patient and educate him about its application in therapy. This stage is particularly important when patient has to take multiple medicines, different medicine at different time. This will remove any confusion from patient's mind which might leads to unintentional misuse of medicament. Also pharmacist should educate the patient regarding benefits of the medicine.

5. **Check patients knowledge of taking medicine:** Ask the patient whether he know how to take medicine. Few simple questions from pharmacist will give idea about whether patient knows how to take medicine or not. If patient is well acquainted about taking the medicine it should be appreciated with good words and if pharmacist found that patient does not know anything or know wrong thing then it should be corrected immediately by giving appropriate information and education. Audiovisual aids, computer softwares and films might be used to educate the patient regarding medication. Color coded labels is one of the effective way to educate the patient to take right medicine at right time in right dose. Few follow up question will confirm the pharmacist that patient understood the treatment regimen correctly. Asking question like "at what time of day you plan to take medicine, how will you schedule medicine during daily activity, how you plan to take medicine during working hours, how will you carry medicine while traveling etc". Pharmacist should confirm correctness of information obtained from patient. Any misunderstanding, misconception should be corrected immediately. Pharmacist should be sure that patient agrees to the communication with the pharmacist. Clear idea should be given to the patient regarding refill of prescription.

6. **Check expectation of patients from medicine:** In response to the questions asked by pharmacist, patient's response will give idea to the pharmacist about outcome of patient's expectations from medicine. Pharmacist can anticipate the level of understanding by the patients regarding communication done. Pharmacist should check the correctness of information provided. Correct any misconception and fill any missing information. Pharmacist should be sure to discuss the therapeutic benefits of medication. Patients will have more adherences to the medicine when he knows potential benefits of

the medicine. Patient should also know possibility of occurrence of any drug interaction. This might create some dilemma in the mind of patients regarding safe use of medicine. Offering solution to such drug interaction will reduce dilemma, resolve the problem and relive the patient from anxiety and empower to patient to deals with therapeutic regimen.

7. **Discuss additional information:** Pharmacist should provide additional information to the patients if needed. The need will be assessed depending on the drugs prescribed, patient's status and illness of the patient. The additional information provided should include.
    - Information regarding drug/food interaction, disease status etc.
    - Consequences of missed dose.
    - Therapeutic monitoring information includes improvement in signs and symptoms due to effective working of drug inside body.
    - Prescription refilling information if required.
    - Storage condition of drug.
    - Change in diet pattern, exercise, lifestyle etc.

    Pharmacist must use his professional skill to understand where the information is to be provided or not and if requires to be provided up to what extend it should be provided. Patient should not be overloaded with information otherwise it might create confusion and dilemma and adherence will be reduced.
8. **Any query from patient:** The closing of counseling process start with asking question to the patients regarding query or question in his mind regarding use of medicine. Patients usually do not ask the question unless they are asked to do so. The presence of any query or concern might distract the patient while providing information by pharmacist. The necessary information may be added for unresolved issues.
9. **Check understanding:** It is most critical case during patients counseling. Asking few question on the information passed to patients will give idea about degree at which patient understood the instructions. The question should be asked using skills otherwise patient might feel that he was put on the quiz and everything will go wrong if he answer incorrectly. The

pharmacist should pinpoint critical issues during such questioning. He may also add any information if missed during counseling process.

10. **Close session:** For closing the counseling process, file the written counseling information obtained during entire session. If needed a written matter should be handed over to the patient. Give the patient your contact number and idea about working hours so that he can approach you if needed for any query aside at latter stage. Confirm to the patient when to return for refilling of prescription or follow up to the physician. Convince patient for values of appropriate medication use and for positive outcome of therapy. Thanks patient for sparing valuable time and wish him good luck for speedy recovery from illness.

Compliance, Adherence, Concordance

Compliance is the action, process initiated and completed by the patients related to instructions, commands, requests, directions concerned with use of medicine, diet, rest, exercise, re-appointment etc. For compliance it is expected from patient that he will follow all the instructions, commands, requests and directions given by health care professionals. In compliance it is assumed that patients are motivated and has positive attitude towards cure from diseases. However it was found that the extent to which patients follow these instructions, command, request and direction varies. Patients might be frustrated from illness. The factors that affect therapeutic outcome include the nature of diseases, duration and nature of treatment, properties of medicines, personality of physician, behaviors of health care professional team. Degree to patient follows these instructions for the benefit and positive outcome of health care professional of treatment varies considerably and hence the term compliance might not be appropriate at this situation. The term compliance is more stringent and strict. It compels the patient to follow the direction of health care professionals same as it is. It requires perfection in execution. The disobedience of directions was not considered. However patients do not follow the instructions as perfectly as expected by the meaning of work compliance. This leads to non-compliance. The more appropriate words used in this concerned are adherence of concordance. The other term used for adherence and concordance are patients adherence, medication adherence, patients concordance, medication concordance.

The adherence means extent to which patients follow the instructions, commands, requests, directions and behaviors that coincides with intention of health care professionals. The term adherence, patient adherence, medication adherence are used in same sense. Although compliance is more popular word adherence is more appropriate and now a day widely used in medical practice. The term adherence is preferred over compliance. The term adherence is linkage between treatment given to the patients and its therapeutic outcome. It is immaterial whether the instructions from physician were strictly followed or not. Many time instructions from health care professionals were not strictly followed by patient. The therapeutic outcome might be little affected but not so significantly. The word adherence will be appropriate in such case. Adherence or non-adherence is a result of complex interaction amongst many factors. There will be unique situation for each patient for prediction and determination of adherence. There is no gold standard for measurement of adherence hence it is difficult to measure and conclude the adherence.

While taking treatment for illness, patients has freedom to choose his own physician, but not on the medicine prescribed by the physician. Many time faith of patient on physician, expectation, concerns, fear, problems determines the effectiveness of treatment. In era of 1990s, the term compliance is more popular in therapeutics and do not take in account faith, expectation, fear, concern and problems of the patient. The term concordance is more appropriate when all these factors were taken into account during drug therapy. The issues of unwanted prescription, overtreatment, inappropriate counseling during therapy leads to misunderstanding and affects the therapy. Unwanted prescription leads to non-use of medicine and results in non-compliance and increase cost of treatment. A concordance is the term used to describe the contribution of patients in consultation, prescribing and decision making for illness. All the decisions made were taken in light of necessities, facts, patient's agenda and financial status. Concordance is new approach includes agreement reached after negotiation between patient and health care professional team. It respects all the issues of patient like belief, wishes, determine whether, when and how medicines are taken. The patient himself also contributes in decision making and hence clearly understood about the treatment he is taking. For consequences (good or bad) he is agree and ready to face them as he is one of the contributors in decision making. The concept of concordance is not yet fully understood and implemented. It is applied only in very few super specialty hospitals, where concern and views of patients were taken in account. For example, during angioplasty procedures which stent (non-medicated, medicated, metallic, polymer based) is to be used for removal of arterial blockade, after surgical procedures in which ward (intensive care, special, general) patient is to be kept for observation.

Barriers

Barriers make the process of counseling more challenging. Patients present barriers. Pharmacist has to overcome these barriers using his experience, skill and various techniques. The barriers of counseling are of two types - functional and emotional. Functional barriers refer to difficulty in receiving and understanding of communication provided by pharmacist. It includes illiteracy, language, visual impairment, hearing impairment, non-English speaking patients etc. emotional barriers come in account when patients are in mental stress, emotional status. Such situations interfere with patients listing, understanding, responding ability and thought process. Emotional barriers include anger, worry, sadness, frustration, embarrassment, depression, mental confusion etc. Pharmacist must recognize these barriers and should take an appropriate step in preventing these barriers or implement appropriate strategy to overcome these barriers. Keen observation, past experience, scientific strategy helps pharmacist to overrule the barriers of counseling. Barriers of counseling vary from patient to patients and strategy to be implemented depending on nature of this barrier.

Functional barriers: Functional barriers can be categorized as sensory, language, condition and other barriers. Pharmacist has to overcome each of these barriers differently. Patient with each type of functional barrier has to treat differently.

Patient with visual abnormality can be identified from seeing eye, dark glasses, thick glasses, holding written material very close etc. Pharmacist can use techniques such as using large and bold font for labeling the containers, Braille label, instructions as per size and shape of container of medicine, use of devices such as magnifier etc. Hearing impaired person can be identified from patient's age, presence of hearing aid, use of signing language, loud speech, frequent repetition, unintentional ignorance of questions (due to non-listening), failure to respond to audio signals etc. The suggested measures to overcome barriers include use of low tone, high volume voice during speaking, use of quiet area for counseling, use of sign language, facial expressions and use of pictographic or written material for communication.

Illiteracy of patient, difference in language, foreign speaking patients and comprehension difficulties are the language related barriers in counseling process. Illiterate patients has difficulty in reading, writing often hide their problem and avoid counseling process. Pharmacist might not detect problem quickly and easily. Use of careful verbal communication, recap of information, pictogram labels, video instructions, use of numbers, color and shapes to distinguish medicines can assist patient in counseling in better manner. Patient who could not speak and understand the English or local language is just like illiterate person who is hearing impaired. Patient will have difficulty in understanding verbal as well as written instruction. Patient responds in foreign language which could not be understood by pharmacist. This could create confusion and inappropriate instruction might be passed. The suggested remedy includes use of non-verbal, body language communication, use of simple terminology, pictograms and auxiliary labels for instructions.

Patients with mental retardation, psychiatric illness has difficulty in comprehension of information communicated during counseling. Presence of comprehensive difficulty is not easy to understand by the pharmacist. No significant signs and symptoms are seen from exterior. Clues of such difficulty can be obtained from psychiatric medications prescribed, history and profile of patient, inappropriate behaviors, dressing, response and manners etc. Pharmacist has to pay extra attention towards these patients. Pharmacist's behavior toward this type of patient should be patience, with kindness, extra attentive. Use of rephrases, careful repetition of instruction is must. Reassure patient, use of demonstrations, asking for feedback will assist both patient as well as pharmacist in follow up.

Emotional barriers: For pharmacist it is difficult challenge to deal with emotional patient. Pharmacist may become uncomfortable with emotional patient ignore issues and responds inappropriately. Pharmacist may focus on solving patient's personal issues of becoming emotional rather than focusing on counseling. When pharmacist come to know that patient is in emotional condition he should focus on solving emotional barrier. Implementation of counseling process when patient is in emotional stage will be useless. Use of empathic response, reflective responding, helps pharmacist to overcome emotional barrier of patient. Pharmacist should listen saying of patient both in the form of verbal and nonverbal communications. In addition pharmacist must have strong desire to understand and help patient. Empathic view towards patient will develop a pharmacist-patient relationship. Over the period of time patient believe in pharmacist and listen to him carefully, this improves quality of care provided by pharmacist toward patient.

Pediatric and Geriatric Counseling

The USP pediatric Advisory Panel has developed a guideline for facilitating the activity that helps children to become active participant in their own health care. The guideline entitled *"Ten Guiding Principles for Teaching Children and Adolescent About Medicine"* includes talking to the parents, gradient and children about occurrence of accidental poisoning, preventive measures and what to do if occurs. When children are sufficiently old to understand about medicine, pharmacist should talk directly to the children about why medicine is given and how to use it correctly. Pharmacist should encourage children to ask questions and queries about their illness, treatment, medicine and its correct use.

Geriatric patients are challenging to the health community pharmacist. It is one of the rapidly growing segments of population. Geriatric patients have many functional barriers. Vision and hearing is mostly impaired in geriatric patients. They have difficulty in performing simple tasks during dose measurement and administration. Pouring medicine from bottle in measuring container, filling insulin syringe, applying cream requires free and skilful movement. Retarded muscular activity, stiffness in joint and week muscles leads to difficulty in performing these tasks. Pharmacist should provide additional time to counsel the geriatric patient. More number of prescribed medicines is main problem with geriatric patients. It can be overcome by written instructions. The effective way of counseling geriatric patients is to provide information in small pieces of specific information. Geriatric patients will get difficulty in understanding, and remembering the large integrative information when provided during counseling.

Role of Pharmacist

Traditional role of pharmacist was to collect the raw material necessary for compounding process, preparation of dosage form and dispensing them as per the directions of the medical practitioner. Due to complexity in diseases, availability of large number of drug and formulations ready made from market, pharmacist start dispensing the medicine as per prescriptions. Pharmacist in hospital is last point to the contact with patient and at competent position and can influence the patient to a large extent. Pharmacist is best suitable person at most suitable place in health care management chain to improve patient compliance through counseling. For the effective counseling they have to maintain good communication skill, sound knowledge, awareness about recent trends in therapeutics and updating of recent discoveries about old drugs and information about newly introduced drugs. To a profession of counselor pharmacist should look as a gentle profession.

The role of pharmacist in counseling is to minimize non-compliance. Pharmacist should be able to fill the gap between therapeutic efficacy of medicine and patient. He makes the patient understand better medicine prescribed for illness. Pharmacists also provide information about diseases, severity, medicine, direction in using medicine; suggest change in life style etc. Pharmacist also counsels the patient for follow-up visit and monitors his medication. Pharmacist also takes telephonic follow-up which improves compliance. Automated telephonic reminder system also improves compliance. Pharmacist can demonstrate, educate and train patients for administration of drugs by special techniques like use of insulin pump, insulin pen, inhalers etc. He can explain, communicate and give information to patients. Counseling by pharmacist reduces missing of dosage during therapeutic regimen.

During ward round participation pharmacist can get opportunity to assist other health care professionals to develop comprehensive skill, capacity and counsel the patient to recover from illness. Advice and counseling by pharmacist encourage the patient for medical adherence, compliance through better understanding illness and medication. This will intern enhance the therapeutic efficacy for rapid recovery from illness. In the view of pharmacist, patient compliance and adherence is associated with communication skill of pharmacist and counseling. Using suitable verbal, non-verbal techniques and method, pharmacist can educate patient. Patient can be educated for possible drug-drug interaction and drug-food interactions. Possible remedies to prevent and avoid these interactions. In such case only clinically significant drug interactions should be mentioned. Minor interaction which might not require much significant clinical intervention should not be included in counseling process, otherwise it might create unnecessary confusion and fear about the medication in the mind of patients and this will leads to poor adherence and non-compliance.

To make patient encourage for better health through self diagnosis, prevention of medicine, healthy lifestyle, avoiding cigarette smoking and alcohol drinking etc. pharmacist should ask simple, indirect, positive questions. Pharmacist should make aware the patient about healthy lifestyle, non-drug intervention, and taking drugs as and when required only. Patient should be counsel such that they will choose healthy lifestyle and not life with medicine.

In Indian context leading problem in patient compliance and adherence is lack of knowledge and information regarding medicine and therapeutic regimen. Physicians are too busy with diagnosis and related aspects of disorder. The consultancy rooms of physicians are unsuitable for patients counseling. Prescription is limited to the signing by physician. Patients are physically tired, with full of anxiety and worries about illness and has poor listening capabilities to physician. The pharmacists are busy with dispensing and part of counseling the patient is ignored. Pharmacists during their academics years spend sufficient time in studying various aspects of drugs. He bears thorough knowledge about medicine, their formulations, therapeutics, medicine from natural origin and legal aspects of pharmacotherapy. This promotes the pharmacist to participate in taking challenges in pharmacy practice scenario. The aim of patient education is "Right medicine to the Right Patient at the Right time in a Right dose through the Right route of administration in the Right manner".

In Indian setting medical adherence can be affected by various positive and negative factors. The positive factors that contributes in medical adherence includes good family support during illness, patient care, joint family setup where special care is taken for pediatrics and geriatrics, good patient-doctor relationship, faith of patients on doctor etc. The factors that has negative impact on medical adherence includes illiteracy, lack of knowledge of diseases and its treatment, precaution and care, poor socioeconomic status of patients etc. Less involvement of pharmacist in patients counseling, improper ratio of physician to patient (around 1: 150-200 in rural area) are also major contributing factors for poor adherence. Pharmacist or physician cannot spare sufficient time for patients counseling. Patients do not have medical insurance and their affordability is very low. Pharmacist has to play a major role in such situation through patient education. In India only 5% pharmacists are involved in active patients counseling. On the other hand in countries like USA pharmacist are responsible for counseling of patients and are involved in fulltime counseling process since 1965.

At around 1980's Indian pharmacists become aware about patient's counseling services and their importance. The official publication of Indian Hospital Pharmacist Association contributes for popularization of concept of patients counseling. Govt. Medical College and Hospital, Trivandrum started separate patients counseling centre in 1992 with very few diploma and graduate and post graduate pharmacists as counselors. Now it is 24 hour service providing patient's counseling centre as a separate department. The team members of counselors include research scholars and service of center is well acclimatized. More counseling centers were started in other regions of south Indian hospital and pharmacy institutes. In these counseling centers pharmacist talk one to one with patients during discussion and counseling and ensures that patients understands the directions and assesses need of follow up. Patients were made aware of drug effects, adverse effect (if have significance) and considerable inconvenience if any and remedial action on side effects if necessary. Patients were also educated regarding drug-drug interactions and drug-food interactions and measures to be taken for that.

The important factor adversely affecting promotion of pharmacy counseling services in India is busy pharmacist, overcrowded pharmacy, poor ration of patients to pharmacist (1 pharmacist for around 14 thousand population), lack of time, non-availability of adequate infrastructural facilities for counseling process and absence of skilled and trained staff members with good communication skill, interviewing technique and counseling ability. The majority of pharmacists working in community pharmacy are diploma qualified. Graduate and post graduate pharmacist select pharmaceutical manufacturing companies, research and development or academics as career options. Selection of community or hospital pharmacist as a professional career in graduate and post graduate students is least priority in our country. The diploma students do not have in-depth knowledge so that they can become effective counselor and graduate students do not select it as a profession. The development of Indian pharmacy as a counseling center will be at par with developed countries till enough graduates and post graduate student will not select the patient counselor as profession.

References

A.J. Winfield, R.M.E. Richards (2004). Pharmaceutical Practice, 3rd edition, Churchill Livingstone.

Ames Gross, Sunil Patel (2002). Indian Pharmaceutical, Industry: Market, Regulatory, Import and Investment Regime. Pacific Bridge.

G. Parthasarathi, Karin Nyfort-Hansen, Milap C Nahata (2012). A Textbook of Clinical Pharmacy Practice, Essential Concepts and Skills, 2nd edition Universities Press (India) Private Limited.

Ganachari M.S, Tarun W, Vimala C.L (2011). Initiation & evaluation of patient counseling centre services to out patients in a tertiary care hospital. *Ind J of Pharm Pract* **4(2):** 23-28.

http://usphs.gov/corpslinks /pharmacy/pdf/hist3.pdf (pharmacy history COA 2005; part 3).

Juliet Higdon (2005). Using counseling skills to communicate more effectively. *Journal of the Malta College of Pharmacy Practice* **10:** 36-37.

K.G. Ravikumar, B.D. Miglani (2009). A Textbook of Pharmacy Practice, 1st edition, Career Publications.

Remington (2005). The Science & Practice of Pharmacy, 21st ed, Lippincott Williams & Wilkins.

Sonal Sekhar M, Suja Abraham, Revikumar KG (2008). Emerging Trends in Practice of Patient Counseling - Indian Scenario. *Indian Journal of Pharmacy Practice* **1(1):** 6-13.

Sunera M. Fernando (2011). Communication skills and counseling. *Sri Lanka Journal of Obstetrics and Gynaecology* **33:** 69-71.

Suresh B (2008). Shaping the pharmacy profession. *Indian Journal of Hospital Pharmacy* **45(1):** 4.

CHAPTER 8

Pharmacy Shop

Establishment and Organization

The establishment of the pharmacy shop should be subject to the objective analysis and community need. The answer of question "Does the community really need facility of pharmaceutical services in the area?" must be found out. The question must be analyzed both in a qualitative and quantitative dimensions. Establishment of pharmacy must fulfill the need and services of community in the area. The needs of community must be identified, analyzed, evaluated in various aspects and various alternates available. The pharmacy must be established to fulfill these needs. Perhaps the already established pharmacy services might not be sufficient or not providing services required. These services must be made available in pharmacy to be established. If requirement and its analysis indicates that pharmacy should be established then pharmacist must consider the following questions.

- What should be the legal requirement for establishment of organization?
- What should be the choice of location of pharmacy?
- What facilities to be created and necessary capital to be made available for it.

The establishment of pharmacy could be done as 1. A sole proprietorship, 2. Partnership 3. Corporation/trust or so. The pharmacy established and managed by individual is a sole proprietorship. Individual shall be the owner of all the property of pharmacy and legally that individual will be responsible for all the activity and consequences in that pharmacy. When the resources of one individual is not sufficient to provide the base of establishment of pharmacy then joint ownership of more than one individual shall be considered as a partnership. It will broaden the financial burden but not the legal responsibilities which always lies with pharmacist. Co-ownership can also be effected by establishing formal organization known as corporation. The corporation offers power to stockholders which limits the liability for business. The legal responsibility can be dedicated to individual pharmacist who can be a stockholder or employee of organization.

The population of area, distribution of income, types of physician and competition climate must be seen during selection of site for establishment of pharmacy. Careful consideration must be done for selection of site. Planning, and assembling the necessary predictable capital must be carefully evaluated for the project of establishment of pharmacy. The amount of capital required for successful operation of pharmacy is the function of productivity. Certain asset is required for fixed core necessaries of any pharmacy while some volume is required as moving asset which is regardless of sale and sale volume. The asset required largely depends on scope of operation and volume of sale anticipated. Sufficient amount of cash in hand is required for preopening expenses and operating expenses like license fees, legal fees, utility deposits etc. and the amount of inventory depends on facilities to be created. The cost of furniture and fixtures may also vary depending on facilities created.

Legal Aspect

Till 1930s India depends on the import of drugs. After the First World War, India becomes a depot of substandard, adulterated, and spurious drugs. Late Sir Henry Gidney (MLA) pointed out the case of quinine fraud. A drug enquiry committee was appointed under chairmanship of Colonel R. N. Chopra and as per the report of committee a separate Drug and Cosmetic Act was came into existence. In practice The Drug Act came in to existence in 1940, presently known as The Drug and Cosmetic Act 1940 and Rules, 1945.

Recommendations from committees like Major General Bhatia committee and other committees time to time lead to amendments in act. Some of the major amendments are listed below –

- Repealing and Amending Act, 40 - 1949
- Adaptation of Law Order - 1950

- The Part B State (Laws) Act - 1951
- The Drug Amendment Act, 11 - 1955
- The Drug Amendment Act, 35 - 1960
- The Drug Amendment Act, 21 - 1962
- The Drug Amendment Act, 13 - 1964
- The Drug Amendment Act, 19 - 1972
- The Drug Amendment Act, 68 - 1982
- The Drug Amendment Act, 71 - 1986
- The Drug Price Control Order - 1995

The Drugs and Cosmetics Act 1940 and Rules, 1945 was framed for regulation of import, manufacturing, sale of drugs and cosmetics in India. The objective of the act is to maintain minimum standards in drugs and cosmetics so that quality product will be available for patients and consumers. The act provides detailed guidelines for research, manufacturing, distribution, retailing and pharmacists working in hospitals. The act provides exhaustive detailing about setup with norms and compliance. The objective of act is self regulation. It gives regulatory authority effective tool to regulate quality management. To the regulatory authority, act gives authorization of licensing, inspection, and power to assess extend of compliance of the facilities.

The Schedule N of The Drugs and Cosmetics Act 1940 and Rules, 1945 gives detailing about list of minimum equipments required for efficient running of pharmacy. Rule 64 of the Act gives details about various conditions to be satisfied before license is granted for sell, stock, exhibit of sale. Rule 65 of the Act specifies various general conditions to be followed in the pharmacy shop (Conditions for License). Rule 65 (A) of the Act gives additional information to be furnished by an applicant for license or a licensee to the licensing authority.

Schedule N

Schedule N of The Drugs and Cosmetics Act 1940 and Rules, 1945 comprises of list of minimum equipments for effective running of a pharmacy store. It includes infrastructural, furniture, apparatus and other facilities. The drug store should bear a name "Pharmacy" in-front of shop. The area of pharmacy should be separated from other area available for other private or business purpose. The area should be properly constructed, ventilated, dry, and of sufficient size to allow proper storage of medicine in stock. A separate area for medicines and poisons should be allocated and should be clearly visible. The area of dispensing should not be less than 6 square meter for one working pharmacist and additional 2 square meters for each additional working pharmacist in the dispensary. The height of drug store should be minimum 2.5 meters. The flooring of pharmacy should be washable and smooth. Walls should be cement plastered, oil painted or tiled so that surface can be maintained smooth, durable and washable devoid of crack and crevices. The pharmacy should be provided with sufficient supply of potable water. The dispensing area in pharmacy should be separate from other pharmacy area and with barrier so that patients and other customers can not have admission in that area.

The furniture and apparatus for the pharmacy should be procured and installed such that it should fulfill the need and demand of the activity intended, size and requirement of establishment. Drugs, chemicals and medicines should be stored as per their property or therapeutic class, or company wise. Drawers, compartments, shelves, glasses can be used to keep the drugs and medicine containers and packs of different size and shape. The order of placing medicine should be in alphabetically or dosage form wise or company wise. The arrangement should be close and tight so as to prevent entry of dust. Each container should bear labeling of proper size as per Pharmacopoeias so that it can be read easily. The top surface of dispensing area should be provided with appropriate surface area suitable for washing and cleanliness. The surface should be preferably made of stainless steel, laminated or plastic. A separate arrangement of cupboard with lock and key should be provided for storage of poisons and should be clearly marked as "POISON" in red letters with white background. The containers used for storage of concentrated solutions should have special label and marked as "To be diluted". The pharmacy must be provided with apparatus and books necessary for dispensing of official preparations and prescriptions. The apparatus consists of following items –

- Beakers of various size (Lipped and assorted)
- Corks of various size and shape, tapers
- Counter balance with 3 kg capacity and 1 gm sensitivity

- Dispensing balance with 30 mg sensitivity
- Filter papers
- Glass funnels of various sizes
- Glass stirring rod
- Graduated pipettes of various capacities (2, 5 and 10 ml)
- Litmus paper (red and blue)
- Measuring cylinders of various capacities (10, 25, 100 and 500 ml)
- Metric weights (1 mg to 100 gm)
- Mortars and pestles made of glass, porcelain and Wedgwood
- Ointment pot with Bakelite or suitable caps
- Pill boxes *
- Pill finisher boxwood *
- Pill machine *
- Porcelain evaporating dish
- Porcelain ointment slab
- Prescription bottle
- Retort iron stand with rings
- Rubber stamp and pad
- Rubber, vulcanite and stainless steel spatulas
- Scissors
- Spirit lamp
- Suppository mould *
- Thermometer (00 to 200 deg. Centigrade)
- Tripod stand
- Watch glasses
- Water bath
- Water distillation still (for eye drop and eye lotion preparation)
- Wire gauze

(* items required and should be provided when intended to dispense pills and suppositories). The list of books required in pharmacy comprises of –

- The Indian Pharmacopoeia (Latest edition)
- National Formulary of India (Latest edition)
- The Drugs and Cosmetics Act, 1940 and rules there under 1945
- The Pharmacy Act, 1948
- Narcotic and Psychotropic substances Act 1985
- Various amendments their after of various Acts and Rules
- Drug Price Control Order

All the activities in the pharmacy must be conducted under the continuous supervision of a Registered Pharmacist and his name and certificate of registration should be displayed noticeably in the pharmacy. During all the activities in the pharmacy, pharmacist should always wear a clean white overcoat. All the things in the pharmacy should be properly kept and everything shall be in good order and clean. All the records and registers should be maintained as per laws and rules. The containers taken out for compounding, dispensing from the poison cupboard should be replaced therein immediately after use and cupboard should be locked immediately. The keys of cupboard should be kept in personal custody of responsible person. Medicines dispensed and supplied should have label confirming to the provision of law in force at that time.

All of above requirement as per the schedule N of The Drugs and Cosmetics Act, 1940 and Rules, 1945 are subject to modification as per the services and facilities created by pharmacy. It is also at the discretion of licensing authority. As per the opinion of licensing authority, the facility created should be as regards to the nature of drug dispensed, compounded and prepared by the licensee. It is the discretionary power of licensing authority to relax the above requirement or to impose additional requirement as per the circumstances of particular case. The decision of licensing authority in this regard is always considered to be final.

Rule 64: Rule 64 (1) under The Drugs and Cosmetic Act, 1940 and Rules, 1945 includes various conditions to be satisfied before a license in form 20, 20-B, 20-F, 20-G, 21 or 21-B for granting approval or renewal of license for sale, stock, exhibit or offer for sale or distribute the drugs (retail and wholesale). These licenses should not be granted or renewed to any person unless authority empowered to grant the license satisfy that the pharmacy to which the license is granted or renewed is adequately equipped for various conditions of storage, accommodation, preservation of the drugs and medicine. The registered pharmacist who will be in charge of pharmacy in the opinion of licensing authority is competent to sale, distribute and preserve the drugs and medicine.

The license to the pharmacy in the form no. 20 and 21(Retail Pharmacy) should not be granted or renewed unless licensing authority satisfies that the prescribed requirements for a pharmacy as per Schedule N have been complied. The license in form 20-F shall be granted or renewed only in the area where pharmacy is not operating. Such license in Form 20-F may be granted to chemist or druggist. The licensing authority must satisfy that for retail Pharmacy, the allotted area should be not less than 10 sq.m.

Rule 64 (2) under The Drugs and Cosmetics Act, 1940 and Rules, 1945 indicates that in granting or renewing the license under sub-rule 64 (1) as above, the licensing authority is empowered to grant or renew the license during the period of 3 years immediately preceding and to the occupancy, trade or business ordinarily carried out on by such application during the period. The licensing authority may refuse to grant or renew the license to applicant or licensee who has been convicted of an offence under the Act or Rule, or licensing authority can cancel or suspend the license granted or renewed under Act and Rule to the person who is not fit for grant or renew of license. Such order of refusal, cancellation or suspension must be communicated to the licensee as soon as possible.

In respect of application for the grant of license in form 20-B or 21-B or both, the licensing authority must satisfy that the pharmacy to which the license is granted or renewed must have area not less than 10 square meters and the competent person in charge of whole sale pharmacy must be registered pharmacist or passed matriculate or equivalent examination and having at least four years of experience in dealing with sales of drugs or having degree from recognized university with one year experience in dealing with sales of drugs.

Rule 65: Rule 65 of The Drugs and Cosmetic Act 1940 and Rules, 1945 prescribed various conditions of licenses. Various license in forms mentioned in Rule 64 shall be subjected to the condition stated herewith.

1. In the pharmacy any drug must be prepared, compounded or dispensed under direct and personal supervision of registered pharmacist only.
2. Other than whole sale, supply of drugs and medicines on the prescription of registered medical practitioner must be effected under direct and personal supervision of registered pharmacist only.
3. Other than those drugs which are specified under category of schedule X, supply of drugs on the prescription of registered medical practitioner at the time of supply must be recorded in the register specially prepared for the same. The serial number of that register must be mentioned on the prescription.

   If the drugs and medicines are not compounded in pharmacy and supplied in original container as it is, then particulars must be entered in cash or credit memo book. If the medicine is supplied on the prescription of registered medical practitioner on previous occasion, a new entry of such dispensing must be made in the register with all the details of new dispensing and reference number of previous dispensing. It is not necessary to record all the details in the register or cash/credit memo if 1. Such supply of drugs is against prescription under the Employee of State Insurance Scheme 2. Any drug other than mentioned in schedule C or H if it is supplied in original, unopened container of manufacturer. The prescription must be duly stamped at the time of supply with name of supplier and date.

   The option to maintain prescription register or a cash memo or credit memo book in respect of drugs and medicines supplied in original container of manufacturer must be made to the licensing authority at the time of granting or renewal of license of retail. Licensing authority may ask licensee to maintain record in prescribed register, if satisfy that the entries made in carbon copy of cash or credit memo are not legible.
4. Supply of drugs by retail other than prescription, specified in schedule C must be recorded in register specially maintained for that purpose. The serial number of the register must be entered in cash memo. The entries in cash/credit memo must

be retained by licensee and these entries must be in legible manner. The option of maintaining register or cash memo must be informed to licensing authority in written during application of grant or renewal of license to sale by retail. Licensing authority may ask licensee to maintain a register if it satisfy that the entries in the carbon copy of cash/credit memo are not legible. Record of purchase of drug intended for sale by retail must be maintained by licensee along with purchase bills including cash/credit memo (bills with serial numbers) in chronological order.

5. Supply of drugs by wholesale must be made against cash/credit memo bearing name and address of licensee and his license number under The Drugs and Cosmetics Act 1940 subject to the fulfillment of other conditions of rule. The particulars must include date of sale, name and address of licensee to whom drugs are sold and his license number, name of drug, quantity and batch number, name of manufacturer and signature of competent person under whose supervision the sale was effected. In case of sale to authority purchasing on behalf of Government, hospital, medical education or research institute the name of authority must be mentioned instead of name of licensee. Carbon copy of cash/credit memo must be preserved as a record for the period of not less than three years from the date of sale.

   The record of resale or intended for wholesale must be maintained by licensee and such record should have date of purchase, name and address and license number, name of drug, quantity and batch number, name of manufacturer of the drug. Purchase bill including cash or credit memo must be serially numbered and maintained in chronological order by licensee.

6. Licensee must produce all the registers and records maintain under the Rules for the inspection by the inspectors appointed under the Act. Licensee must provide all the information required for the purpose of ascertain that the provision of Act and Rules there under has been observed.

7. Except, where otherwise mentioned in the Rule, all the registers, records maintained under these Rules must be preserved for the period of not less than two years from the date of last entry in the record.

8. Anything which is not withstanding with this Rule shall not to be necessary to record any particulars in the register specially maintained for the purpose as per the Rule and other law for the time being in force.
9. Substances mentioned in the schedule H or Schedule X shall not be sold by retail on or in accordance with the registered medical practitioner. In case of schedule X drugs, the prescription must be in duplicate and one copy of which must be retained and preserved by licensee for the period of 2 years after sale of drug.
10. The prescription for the above clause 9 must be in writing and signed by the person giving it and date. It should also specify name and address of the person for whom treatment is given, indicating total number of medicine to be supplied and dose to be taken.
11. The person dispensing the prescription containing drugs specified in schedule H and schedule X must comply with the following requirement in addition to the requirement of the Rule.
    (a) The prescription must not be dispensed more than once unless stated by the prescriber that the prescription may be dispensed more than once.
    (b) If prescription contains direction for number of times of dispensing and intervals then dispensing must be done accordance with directions.
    (c) At the time of dispensing, pharmacist must note on the prescription above the signature of prescriber, name and address of seller and date on which prescription is dispensed.

    As per the clause 11-a no person dispensing the prescription containing substances specified in Schedule H or Schedule X supply other preparation containing same substance or in lieu thereof (No substitution).
12. The substances specified in Schedule X kept in pharmacy must be stored under lock and key cupboard or drawer reserved solely for the storage of these substances or separated from other section of pharmacy and to which only responsible person has access.

13. This clause was omitted by G.S.R. 462(E), dt. 22-6-1982 (w.e.f. 22-6-1982)

14. This clause was omitted by G.S.R. 462(E), dt. 22-6-1982 (w.e.f. 22-6-1982)

15. As per the rule and schedule the description, name, label of shop must be put as "Drug Store" by licensees who do not requires having services of registered pharmacist.

    As per the rule and schedule the description, name, label of shop must be put as "Chemist and Druggist" by licensees who do requires and employ the services of registered pharmacist but do not maintain the pharmacy for compounding against prescription.

    As per the rule and schedule the description, name, label of shop must be put as "Pharmacy", "Pharmacist", "Dispensing Chemist". "Pharmaceutical Chemist" by licensees who do require and employs the services of registered pharmacist and maintain the pharmacy for compounding against prescription.

    "Registered Pharmacist" means a person or individual who is registered as a pharmacist as per definition in clause (i) of Section (2) of the Pharmacy Act 1948 (Act 8 of 1948), provided that the provision of sub-clause (i) shall not apply to those who are already provided as "qualified pharmacist" by the licensing authority on or before 31st December 1969.

    Date of expiry of potency means the date that is recorded on the container label or wrapper as the date up to which the substance may be expected to retain a potency not less than or not to acquire a toxicity greater than that required or permitted by the prescribed test.

16. The licensee in his pharmacy should maintain an Inspection Book in form No. 35 to enable an inspector to record his impression and the defects noticed.

17. No drug shall be sold, stocked by the licensee in pharmacy after the date of expiry of potency recorded on its container, label or wrapper or in violation of any statement or direction recorded on such container, label or wrapper.

    Any such expiration drug, licensee may stock or keep with him only if manufacturer or his representative has policy of withdrawal, reimbursement or disposal of the expired drugs or products. All such withdrawal, reimbursement or disposal are subjected to condition that stock of such expired drugs must be stored separately from the trade stock and all such expired drugs that are kept in packages, containers or cartons which are labeled prominently as "NOT FOR SALE".

18. The drugs which are intended for distribution as a free sample to the medical profession shall not be stocked or sold by the licensee in the pharmacy. Such drugs have a label on the container as per the clause (ix) of sub-rule (1) of Rule 96. The other category of drugs included are drugs meant for consumption by the employees State Insurance Corporation, the Central Government Health Scheme, the Government Medical Stores Depots, the Arm Force Medical Stores and other Government institutes. The drugs have distinguishing marks or any inscription on label of the container indicating the purpose.

    This above clause will not be applicable to the licensee who is appointed as approved pharmacist, chemist or druggist by the State Government under the Employee's State Insurance Scheme, or has been appointed as authorized agent/distributor by the manufacturer manufacturing the drugs meant for consumption by the Central Government Health Scheme, the Government Medical Stores Depots, the Arm Force Medical Stores and other Government institutes, or has been appointed and authorized by the manufacturer for storing of free samples meant for distribution to the medical professionals. The stock of such free sample must be stored separately from the trade stock and separate record of stock received and distributed must be maintained by the licensee.

19. The retail supply of any drug in an envelope or any other suitable container other than one in which the manufacturer has marketed the drug shall be made only by the dealer who in turn takes the services of registered pharmacist and such supply shall be made under the direct supervision of registered pharmacist only. The label of such containers must show the particulars indicating name of drug, quantity supplied, name and address of dealer.

20. The drugs and medicines intended for animal use should be kept in pharmacy shall bear label "NOT FOR HUMAN USE".

Such medicine must be stored in cupboard or drawer reserved solely for the storage of veterinary drugs or in a part of pharmacy separated from area where patients and customer does not have access. Should have animal picture on the label and also on the storage cupboard where these drugs have been stored so that they can be identified and located.

21. At the time of supply, the drugs specified in Schedule X must be recorded in a bound register, serially numbered and specially maintained for the purpose. Separate page must be allotted for each drug. The particulars entered in such register should have date of transaction, quantity received with name and address of supplier and number of relevant license by supplier, name of drug, quantity supplied, manufacturers name, batch no. and lot no., name and address of patients, purchaser, reference number of prescription, bill no. and date of purchase, signature of person under whose supervision drug is supplied.

Rule 65 (A): Rule 65 A of the Drugs and Cosmetics Act, 1940 and Rules 1945 includes additional information to be furnished by an applicant for license of a licensee to the licensing authority. The applicant who applies for grant of license should furnish the information to the licensing authority before grant of license or during the period of license in force the entire relevant documentary evidences indicating ownership, occupation on rent or other basis of the pharmacy specified in his application for the license or his license granted. These documents must be for the purpose of verification of correctness of the statement made by the applicant or licensee while applying or after obtaining a license as the case may be.

Requirement

Infrastructure: The location of drug store/pharmacy should be such that it must be acceptable to all stake holders. The location should have approach road to bring the vehicle who will supply medicines and goods directly very near to the shop. The local area of shop should be planted with trees to provide shade and offset high temperature. Building of store should be done on raised platform or foundation to allow rain water to drain away from store and does not accumulate near or inside the store. There should be proper fencing to the premise besides the controlled access to the double locking doors. The pharmacy should have suitable fire protection devoice. Fire extinguisher should be inspected every 2 to 3 months and should be serviced and charged at least every 12 months. Smoke detectors must be placed in and checked every 2 to 3 month. Emergency exit must be marked clearly and checked regularly for its functioning and accessibility. The inside and outside building of the pharmacy must be regularly inspected for cleanliness, evidence of pests. Food should not be kept or left inside the pharmacy as it invites the rodents. The interior must be kept dry and clean.

The infrastructure required for drug store/pharmacy should comprise of minimum following requirement.

- Adequate storage facility must be created in shop for storage and handling of medicines. The requirement of space depends on quantity of supply received, length of stay of medicine inside the shop etc.
- In large facilities special cold rooms can be created where as in small drug stores freezers or refrigerators can be used.
- The location and design of pharmacy should ensure maximum air circulation to avoid accumulation of fumes and gases. Exhaust fan, high and wide windows should be provided to ensure proper temperature and humidity control.
- Proper drainage should be provided for water accumulated on roof and floor. Roof must be extended on windows to give extra protection from rain and direct sunlight. Double sealing should be installed to provide insulation. The walls and floor should be smooth and easy for cleaning. Construction should be of brick or concrete.
- The door of shop must be wide enough for easy and free movement of supplied material and strong enough to provide adequate protection.
- As far as possible natural light must be used. Use of florescent or incandescent lighting must be avoided as they have adverse effect on stability of certain medicinal products.

- Cupboards and shelves must be provided to keep the specific products free from dust and light. Some cupboards must have lock and key arrangement for storage of restricted medicines.

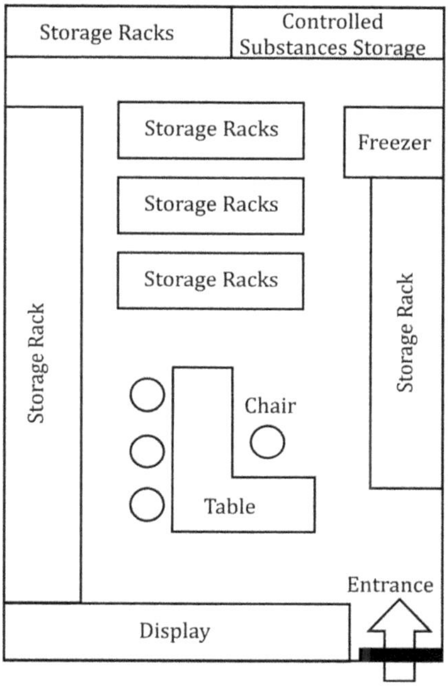

Retail pharmacy shop

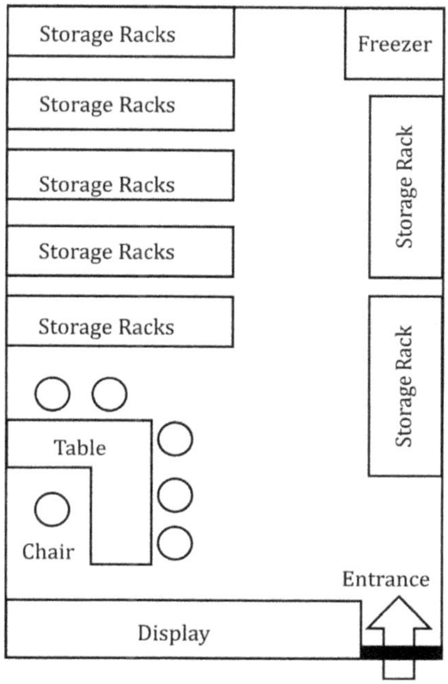

Wholesale pharmacy shop

Drug Information System (DIS): The drug information system is an artificial system which consists of peoples, hardware, software, books, journals and other resources. The aim of DIS is to collect timely, correct, processing, storage, transmission and provision of information for the activity of organization which might be patient centered or of administrative importance. In management information system the past data can be assessed and utilized for prediction of future, assess the overall situation and decision making.

A pharmacy must have minimum text required for maintaining drug information system. The drug information request must be handled by pharmacist. Pharmacist should select the current literature or reference source for gathering the information. Before delivering the information pharmacist must assure, evaluate and analyzed the relevant drug and information source from current literature. A system of classification and organization must be developed for management of information. Readily accessible filing, cross indexing, must be maintained. Pharmacist must use professional expertise and judgment in processing drug information. Step of information flow includes obtaining necessary background information, interpreting drug information, conducting literature survey, evaluating literature in accurate and unbiased manner, formulating relevant information and communicating the information in verbal or written form. The drug information should be current. The pharmacist should be aware of more and extensive source of information and procedure to access the information.

Computers: Computers are required in all aspects of drug store management from selection of product to usage. Computer system is capable of manipulating text and numbers and also useful in participating in report generation, tables, graphs, newsletters. Along with use of communication device (like LAN, internet, telephone) in association with computer system can be used for exchange and share of information and data. With effective utilization of computer system quality of service can be improved, saves money, promote efficiency. However poorly implemented computer system wastes money, decreases efficiency, distracts attention and requires more time for working.

Computer technology changes very quickly with time. Technology becomes faster, more capable of handling complicated tasks and less expensive. The effectiveness of computer system depends on choice of computer; tools attached to it, effective utilization of these tools and overcome the hurdles of incorporation of computer system in existing setup. There is no definite standard formula for successful computerization of drug store management.

Implementation of computer system help in effective implementation of DIS: 1. Simplifies and speeds up the complex tasks and increases accuracy (by spell-check, calculation, data integration) 2. Help to update and access information quickly 3. Perform automated repetitive task 4. Provide information for management for decision making 5. It allow organization to expand volume and scope of operation 6. Streamlines administrative objectives 7. Generates reports timely without efforts. However computers have some limitations. They cannot assume responsible for making wrong decisions. Computer system cannot define objective, define problem, improve basic data available and make person more organized. If appropriate hardware and software are not procured they will not fulfill the need. Computerization is not a onetime investment, continuous training, support and up gradation is required in hardware and software.

Pharmacy Management

Financial: The extent of effective management of pharmacy depends on ability of generating money from various sources in sufficient quantity. The objective of financial management is to have a maximum rate of returns on the investment made. Financial management not only applies to the cash but also to those material and services that are used to operation of pharmacy.

The costing on drugs in pharmacy consumes around 60% of the total consumable budgets. There can be a saving up to 20% on controlled expenses on drugs. ABC and VED matrix is the most suitable and popular for financial management of medical store. ABC analysis is known as "Always Better Control" used for financial management on material costing. The management based on Pareto's principle of vital few and trivial many. According to Pareto's principle 10% of items consume about 70% of budget (known as Group A item). Around 20% items consumes 20% financial budget (known as Group B item) and remaining 70% items accounts for 10% budget (known as Group C item). As per VED analysis V is for vital items without which pharmacy cannot function, E is essential items without which pharmacy will function but may affect the quality of service and D represents desirable items, unavailability of which will not interfere with function. Combined together ABC and VED matrix can be distributed as AV, BV, CV, AE, BE, CE, AD, BD and CD.

Material: A material management in pharmacy store includes supplier selection, quality assurance, procurement and distribution of material. Supplier should be pre-qualified and during supply they should be monitored through the process to maintain product quality, service reliability, in time delivery. The drugs and material procurement procedures should include all the assurance that the drugs purchased are of high quality and standards. The drug procurement depends on number of factors like estimating quantity of each drug required at given period, assessing cost of drug dosage and resource allocation to each drug dosage form depending on priority and resources. The requisition of drug and dosage form has to give after assessment of need. Good procurement practice comprises of procurement by generic name, limited to essential drug, in bulk, with supplier's qualification from competitive suppliers. The ordered quantity should depend on reliable need, payment and financial mechanism, transparency and procedure, product quality assurance, annual audit.

The primary goal of material management is to maintain steady supply of drugs and facilities need ensuring that the resources are being used in most effective way. A well managed distribution system should: 1. Maintain constant supply of drug, 2. Keep drugs in good condition, 3. Minimizes drug losses due to spoilage and expiry, 4. Rationalized drug storage points, 5. Reduce theft and fraud and providing information for forecasting drug need, 6. Using available transport as efficiently as possible. The distribution cycle begins when drugs were dispatched from manufacturers/suppliers and it ends when drug is consumed and information of consumption is reported back to the procurement unit. The material management system comprises of seven components: 1. Preparation of drug list, 2. Supply, 3. Ordering, 4. Receiving supply, 5. Organizing drug supplied 6. Inventory management and 7. Record keeping.

Storage: The basic concept of organization, management and storage of drug is the ability to locate the supply in store easily from its predetermined location. The principles of storage, organizing and supplies of drug and medicine includes

- Drugs must be stored in original container, similar category (tablets/injection/external preparation etc.) are to be kept on same shelf.
- Medicines are to be ordered in alphabetic order.
- Medicines with short shelf life must be kept at front and dispensed first, it must be ensured that expiry date of medicine must be visible clearly from front side.
- Top shelves should contain dry formulations like tablets, capsules etc., middle selves should contain liquid preparations like liquid orals, injections, ointments etc. and bottom shelves should contain surgical and laboratory items.
- Items must be stored in groups so that can be counted easily.
- Medicines must be kept at least 10 cm above the floor level, 30 cm away from wall and not more than 2.5 meter in height.

- Manufacturer directions must be followed during storage. It is essential to follow the instruction of manufacturer's storage instruction to the extent possible. If not possible then product must be stored in possible suitable condition and dispensed as quickly as possible.
- High value products must be kept in security zone.
- If no specific storage condition is mentioned then it should be stored in dry condition at temperature between 15 to 25 °C and maximum up to 30 °C.
- The storage area must have provision for monitoring room temperature and temperature must be recorded at least once a day at hottest time of day.
- Indian Pharmacopoeia describes storage condition of official substances which are likely to be deteriorated.
  - ***Store frozen***: Vaccines need storage below – 20 °C
  - ***Do not freeze***: To be kept in refrigerator at + 2 to + 8 °C
  - ***Keep cold***: To be stored at temperature not exceeding 8 °C
  - ***Keep cool***: To be stored at temperature 8 to + 25 °C
  - ***Ambient temp.***: Store at room temperature (R.T) 18 - 25 or up to 30 °C
  - ***Protect from moisture***: To be stored in normal humidity at R.T.
  - ***Protect from light***: To be stored in light resistant cupboard/drawer

Inventory: Inventory management of medicine in medical store/pharmacy is the scientific process by which pharmacy is supplied with goods and services in order to provide the services in optimum cost. Proper inventory control will manage the cost balance between shortage and excess stock. Without proper control of inventory management a serious problems can precipitate related to revenue generation, customer's satisfaction in terms of non-availability of medicine or dispensing of near to expiry drugs. Inventory control involves process of decision as to when, what and how much of each item is to be kept in stock, minimization of ineffective stock and optimizing the various causes associated with inventories.

To minimize inventory, resources must be utilized most efficiently and effectively. The record of available material must be maintained for maintaining optimal quantity. Ineffective stock must be minimal. Various cost related to inventory must be minimized. Scope of inventory control includes reduced cost, improved service delivery, increased return on investment, improved liquidity, improved service conditions, improved efficiency of man and machine and improved patient's satisfaction.

Staff: An important aspect for effective operation of pharmacy is well-conceived program of staff/personal management. The selection and maintenance of personals must be given top priority. Proper selection, training and maintenance of employee will create a unique personal and care taking atmosphere in the pharmacy. Each employee in pharmacy represents the shop to physician, patients and suppliers. The success and failure of pharmacy also depends on the nature, behavior and knowledge component of employee. In view of this many pharmacy managers look for good personal administration and management skills. Seasonal variation in work load may alter the number of employee for retailing activity. It may require concentrating of activity during particular period of time in weeks, days or even certain hours of the day. The blend of part time and full time employee should be managed during such rush hours. Extensive use of part time employee without previous work experience, knowledge and economic values of the services may leads to the loss in terms of services or financials. Such part time employee may also require prior training to inculcate the work culture and nature of responsibility in them. Period content updating and training is also essential for full time employee and to the administrator also.

The full time or part time employee are in continuous contact with public, patients, physicians and other stake holders so they must be of at least average intelligence, good appearance and having a acceptable personality. The good staff will always be motivated, encouraged for cleanliness, contributes for good staff morale.

Drug Distribution

A study conducted by Al Hamarneh in 2011 concludes that the major activity of hospital pharmacist is focused either on drug or drug distribution. Only minor responsibility is related to patients centered activity. In 1992 Strand stated that pharmacy services requires timely, accurate drug distribution, timely and complete patients data, comprehensive and current drug information and documentation.

The fundamentals of Strand remain same till date. The basic element of pharmacy is timely and accurate drug distribution. The objective of drug distribution service is to deliver a right medicine to right patient in right presentation in a right dose at the right time at the right cost. The effectiveness of distribution of drug is assessed in terms of accuracy, appropriateness and efficacy. The distribution system of medicine provide health care facilities to the patients in a timely manner as per need, with lowest possible errors, in minimal cost, minimal wastage, minimal medicinal diversion, should provide data of medicine and usage pattern of medicine.

The distribution systems of medicine in Indian market govern by various agencies. It includes four to five layer structures comprising of manufacturer, clearing and forwarding agencies, depots, super stockist, stockist, wholesalers and retailers. Some distribution system follows complete path while other follows small number of steps in the path through which drug flows. The flow of drug from one layer to other was initially influence by two tier tax structure, central sale tax (CST) and local sale tax (LTC). Later on this taxation system was replaced slowly by value added tax system (VAT).

Stockist does the marketing of products of around 6 to 8 pharmaceutical companies. There are very few stockists which market product of more than 50 companies. Mergers and acquisition of companies vary this number. Stockist of same company compete with each other although they market same product of same company and such stockist have their own chain of market and visiting salesman. Stockist got around 8 to 10 percent of profit margin on their sale. The next step of marketing chain is large number of retailers, we termed by different names as pharmacist, druggist and chemist etc. Retailers account for 70 to 80 percent of product sale. The remaining is account for hospital supply and distribution. Out of total retail market around 25 to 35 percent retailers are located in rural and small town. Retailers are entitled for around 16 to 20 percent of profit margin. Small independent medical shops dominate the retailing of medicines. The pharmacy chain market is developing in India. Subhiksha started its supermarket-cum-pharmacy shops chains at around 1997 in South India. They have around 170 drug stores and account for 300 crore of turnover. In 2007 Apollo, Lifeken, Medicine Shoppe, CRS health has also started their chain pharmacy stores. Ranbaxy, Fortis Healthcare, Zuellig Pharma, Reliance Dhirubhai Ambani Group also proposed to start such chain pharmacy stores. The One stop shop offers the services including prescription of OTC product, health supplement, health food, alternative medicines like ayurvedic and homeopathic medicines, personal care products, pathology collection centre, home delivery of medicine, prescription reminder services etc. Such chain pharmacy stores tie up with pharmaceutical manufacturer and purchase medicines and goods directly from manufacturer and send to the retailers. The margin of intermediate step skips and leads to reduction in price medicine or better services to the patients in the same cost like free home delivery, patients counseling, prescriber reminder services etc.

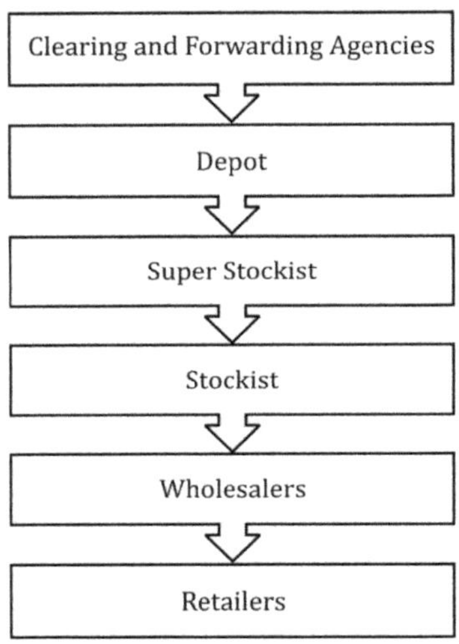

OTC drug distribution: Today's lifestyle is more informed, use more gadgets, fast, facing high stress. Environmental changes, increased pollution, heavy road traffic leads to increased commuting time. Stressful workplace environment put continuous stress on human body. Less exercise, junk food, addictive product to stay alert at job put additional stress. Body expressed all this in the form of psychosomatic disorder like headache, allergy, constipation, common cold, acidity, backache, fatigue etc., and to manage it all over the counter (OTC) drugs were consumed.

Over the counter drugs are also known as non-prescription drugs. These drugs are safe and can be sold by pharmacist without prescription of registered medical practitioner. It includes drugs like vitamin supplements, antacids, paracetamol etc. In recent years the trend of self medication has been increasing with OTC drugs, which are readily available at the pharmacy. In Indian context OTC product has no legal recognition. All the drugs which are not included in the list of prescription drugs are considered as OTC drugs and products. As per the Drugs and Cosmetics Act, the prescription drugs come under two categories Schedule H and Schedule X. The drugs that are under Schedule G require mandatory text on the label "Caution: *It is dangerous to take this preparation except under medical supervision*".

In India import, manufacturing, distribution and sale of drug is regulated by Drugs and Cosmetic Act and its subordinate legislation The Drugs and Cosmetics Rules. The OTC committee of organization of pharmaceutical producers of India (OPPI) is working towards promotion of OTC products. The aim of this committee is to regulate issues related to access of OTC medicine and awareness towards responsibility of self medication. The Drugs and Magic Remedies (Objectionable Advertisement) Act prohibits the misleading advertisement and advertisement which give direct or indirect false impression regarding character of drug, making false claim and claims that are false or misleading in any aspect of the drug/product.

Most of the OTC products are although safe, they are also effective, economic, and readily available. The perceived value of OTC medicine is high. The safe use and effectiveness of OTC product depends on the patient's judgment, diagnosis of disorder and symptoms, information on the label. Incorrect diagnosis, selection of inappropriate medicine, consumption of drug in inadequate dose may leads to no efficacy or toxicity. The pharmacist and pharmacy should engage in legal distribution of drugs. Deemed OTC dispensing should not be practiced. Patient should be interviewed and counseled for the disease condition and appropriate use of medicine. Advertisement of digestives, antacids, cold rub, vitamins, tonics, health supplements, skin treatment products, glucose powder, analgesics etc. type of OTC product can be seen on television and in news papers in India. In the United States out of total pharmaceutical market around 26% of the market share is of OTC products. In India this share is around 27%.

The study concludes that the information given on the outer box of medicine is common source of information for all users. Users expect the simple instructions about the OTC product on the box. Package inserts contain detailed information but very few users refer this information. Warnings and cautions are easily overlooked. Hence while dispensing OTC product, pharmacist should do proper patients counseling.

Outdoor patient distribution: An outdoor patient is the patients who receive medicine on the order of prescription of the physician. Outdoor patient might be non-hospitalized patient or a patient who is to be discharged from hospital after a period of admission and does not require to be admitted in the hospital but require taking a medicine for some period of time for completion of therapeutic regimen. Physician gives him a prescription and advice to take a medicine for a specific period of time. The pharmacist has to dispense drugs as per the prescription of the physician. The patients receive the medicines and take them home with him. Patient takes these medicines as per the advice and instructions of the physician. Pharmacist has to counsel the patient for regular administration of drug. Pharmacist should also advice patients various aspects of medicines like frequency of dose, appropriate storage, predicted side effects etc. In Indian contest this area is well developed and many time managed by less qualified pharmacist. Hospital may also provide medicines to the outdoor patients as an emergency dispensing. This dispensing is done under supervision of medical practitioner and who is member of hospital medical staff. Designated registered nurse also can dispense medicine if prescription is authorized by registered medical practitioner.

Indoor patient distribution: The medicine for indoor patients is prescribed by physician, dispenses by pharmacist and nursing staff administers to the patients who are hospitalized. Dispensing is done by adopting various techniques like plate, envelop, basket system. Unit dose dispensing has gained the importance and popularity, now days because the dose which is to be administered is only dispensed and no unnecessary stocking of drug is done at the bed side of the patient. Computerized system is widely used in unit dose dispensing system. The computerized system is used by pharmacist to keep the record and profile of ambulatory patient, perpetual inventory, charge and non-charge on floor stock, drug related information etc. In Indian context the computerized maintenance of medication for indoor patients is still in budding stage.

Hospital supply: The medicines which are consumed most are many times procured by the hospital in large quantity. Minimal quantity of drugs may be stocked in the patients care area to meet the immediate therapeutic need of patients. Intravenous admixtures, salines, IV sets, bandages etc. are required in many hospitals in very large quantity. Stock of such drugs and appliances is kept at floor level. Pharmacy has to supply such drugs in bulk quantity. Most of the time, such drugs are utilized for indoor patients.

Many hospitals faced a problem of inefficient medication distribution system, leading to inappropriate dispensing, dispensing with errors, involvement of large numbers of pharmacist in dispensing process etc. Managing the inventory of medicine on daily basis is also a tedious task. Automated drug distribution system in hospital is the solution for all these, comprises of computerized automated coding and dispensing of medicaments. Improved inventory management and automation in inventory control helps in management, prediction of sale and exhaust of stock of medicine. Inventory functions were made faster and easier in real time. It is possible to search and locate lot number and expiration of medicine.

References

Ajith Paninchukunnath (2007). OTC Drug Marketing – Global Trends and Indian Experiences, International Marketing Conference on Marketing & Society. 8-10 April, *IIMK* 363-370.

Al Hamarneh YN, Rosenthal M, McElnay JC, Tsuyuki RT (2011). Pharmacists' perceptions of their professional role: insights into hospital pharmacy culture. *Can J Hosp Pharm* **64(1):** 31-35.

Deshpande S.W, Gandhi Nilesh (2007). Drugs and Cosmetics Act, 1940 and Rules, 1945, 4th ed, Susmit Publisher, Mumbai.

Gopalakrishnan P, Sundaresan M (1985). Material management: An integrated approach, 1st ed, New Delhi: Prentice Hall of India Pvt. Ltd.

Gupta S, Kant S (2000). Hospital stores management: An integrated approach, 1st ed, New Delhi : Jaypee Bros Medical Publishers Pvt. Ltd.

Gupta VK, Gupta CD, Patel JR (2013). Assessment of awareness and attitude towards over-the-counter (OTC) drugs amongst urban population: A questionnaire based study. *RJPBCS* **3(2):** 1037-1041.

Kant S, Pandaw CS, Nath LM (1997). A management technique for effective management of medical store in hospitals. *J Acad Hosp Adm* **89:** 41-7.

Kiyomi Sadamoto, Yutaka Higashimata, Masaru Mizoguchi, Takahiro Yamanouchi, Noriyuki Kinoshita, and Tsuyoshi Saeki (2012). Expected

Information of Users for the OTC Drugs in Japan. *Adv Pharmacoepidem Drug Safety* 1-3.

Lt Col R Gupta, Col K K Gupta, Brig B R Jain, Maj Gen R K Garg (2007). ABC and VED analysis in medical store inventory. *MJAFI* **63:** 4.

Pharmaceutical Distribution system in India, The centre for International Public health policy, working paper 1a, prepared for workshop on "Tracing pharmaceutical in South Asia" 2-3 July 2007, University of Edinburg.

Pillans PI, Conry I, Gie BE (1992). Drug cost containment at a large teaching hospital. *Pharmacoeconomics* **1:** 377-82.

Practice standards (2006), SHPA standards of practice for the distribution of medicines in Australian hospitals. *J Pharm Pract Res* **36(2):** 25-1 – 25-7.

Reading material on Drug store management and rational drug use for medical officers, nurses and pharmacist, State Institute of health and Family welfare, Rajastan (Dec. 2010).

Regis Vaillancourt (2011). Pharmacist: The guardian of safe medication use. *JCPH* **64:** 1-6.

Remington (2005). The Science &Practice of Pharmacy, 21st ed, Lippincott Williams & Wilkins.

Strand LM, Cipolle RJ, Morley PC (1992). Pharmaceutical care: an introduction. Kalamazoo (MI): The Upjohn Company.

Toshio Awahya *et al.,* (2005). Automation in drug inventory management saves personnel time and budget. *Yakuga Zasshi* **125(5):** 427-432.

CHAPTER 9

Professional Ethics

Definition

The services of pharmacist are highly valued. There is always expectation of good services in ethical manner. The prime responsibility of pharmacist is to preserve these services in ethical manner. To preserve the services, maintaining only quality and standards are not enough. Along with it, pharmacist has to look after the ethical concerns of the services also. In order to maintain quality and standards, ethics should not be compromised.

Traditions or beliefs that have been evolved over several years and centuries in society deciding or concerning with right and wrong conducts is called as morality. Justification of action and practice in specific situation is concerned with ethics. It is philosophical reflection on moral of life and principles embedded in it. Ethics generally deals with reasoning process. Morality can be thought of as a social institution that has a history and a code of conduct that are implicit or explicit about how people ought to behave. Domain of inquiry, a discipline in which matter of right and wrong, good or evil, virtue and vice and systematically examined is referred as ethics. In contrast morality refers to patterns of thought and action actually operated in day to day life rather than discipline. In this concerned morality is discipline of ethics. The morality of pharmacist is patterns of thought and action operated in day to day working as a professional pharmacist and discipline in this moral thought and action is pharmacist's professional ethics.

For pharmacist ethics is set of values that guide him in his professional life. It consists of right conducts and good life. It is bigger than analysis of what is right and wrong. For the pharmacist central point of ethics is "good life and life worth living for patients".

Ethics controls what we think, interpret to make the decision, take action and also affect the process of learning. Universal behaviors cannot be controlled by single ethics. Hence ethical issues for pharmacist vary from country to country. Ethics is matter of balancing between rights versus right. That is deciding the priority between two right things. Philosophy of ethics applicable to real life situation is applied ethics. It involves setting of standards.

In all ethics can be defined as "Careful, systematic inquiry in to the nature of morality, guidelines or standards that give meaning and direction to community". It is concerned with duties and obligations of pharmacist towards patient and himself.

Code of Ethics

Pharmacist is the key member of health care service provider team. It helps patient for making the best use of medicine. American Pharmacists Association has prepared and published the code of ethics. These ethics forms principles and fundamental basis of roles and responsibilities of pharmacist. These ethics guides pharmacist for his relationship with patient, health care professionals and society. These codes of ethics were originally published in "Code of Ethics for Pharmacists" in American Journal of Health-system Pharmacist (1995), 52: 2131, by American Society of Health System Pharmacists Inc. These eight codes describe relationship of pharmacist with patients, professional relationship and relationship with colleagues, services to community, society and health resources. It includes –

Relationship with Patient

This code of ethics is about the conventional relationship of pharmacist with patient. The pharmacist should respect this conventional relationship. The relationship between pharmacist and patient has covenant means. Pharmacist has moral responsibility in response to the gift of trust received from patient and society. In response to this gift, morally pharmacist should provide individual optimum benefit from the medicine prescribed for illness. Pharmacist should maintain the trust and welfare of patients. Pharmacist should avoid conflict of interest and first consider the patient's health and well-being.

Patients Care

This ethic talk about providing good for every patient in caring, sympathetic and in confidential manner. Patient is centre point of health care management system. Everything happened in health care should be patient centered. Pharmacist is always concerned with well-being of patients at the center of health care system. Pharmacist is always concerned with the fulfillment of needs of patient as demanded by patients or defined by the physician. Pharmacist must dedicate his services in protection of dignity of patient. Pharmacist should focus on providing services to the patients with caring attitude and sympathetic spirit. The services should be provided to patient in private and confidential manner. Pharmacist must respect patient's right of privacy and confidentiality. Pharmacist must do utmost for protection of patient's confidentiality and share the patient's information with other health care professional team members. Unless provided by law, pharmacist should not disclose patient's information without consent of patient. Pharmacist should maintain confidentiality in creating, storing, accessing, transferring and disposing of confidential information.

Autonomy and Dignity of Patients

Pharmacist should respect autonomy and dignity for each patient. Patient has the right to choose his physician and health care taker. Pharmacist should respect the right of patient of self determination and should encourage for participating in decision making about their health. The pharmacist should communicate with patient in language and words that can be easily understandable. All pharmacists should respect and take into account the cultural and personal differences between patients. Pharmacist should utilize professional judgment to protect interest of patients in achieving their selected health outcome. Pharmacist should assist patient in making decisions by providing information about benefits and risks of medicine. Here the term risk is used to define frequent adverse effects. Pharmacist should accept the patient's right to accept or refuse health related recommendations. Pharmacist should obtain voluntary consent from patient prior to provision of pharmacy services. The act of pharmacist should be in the interest of patient benefit and not for exploitation in interest of personal, physical, emotional, financial, social or sexual gain.

Honesty and Integrity in Profession

In his professional career pharmacist should act with honesty and integrity. It is the responsibility of pharmacist to tell the patients the truth with conviction of conscience about illness and medicine prescribed. It is prevented by physician then he should not be. Pharmacist should avoid practice that will discriminate one patient from other. Behaviors of pharmacist also should not discriminate patients. His professional judgment and action should comprise of dedicated action to the best of patient's interest. Pharmacist should provide information to patients in understandable and sensitive manner. Pharmacist should work with ethics, honesty and integrity to support public trust confidence in the profession. Pharmacist must report to appropriate legal authority about unethical practices, incompetency by colleagues or other health care professional. Pharmacist should support advancement in quality of pharmacy services and care. Pharmacist should not participate or involved in dishonesty, fraud, misrepresentation, unethical work and illegal behaviors. Pharmacist should confirm to legal and professional norms which will be used for the integrity and dignity of profession. Pharmacist must use truth, accurate, full, non-deceptive information and should not make false claims in community training programs or marketing. Pharmacist should keep business and professional relationship with only those companies, organization or parties which follow and comply code of ethics and interest of standards.

Professional Competency

Pharmacist must maintain professional competency. Pharmacist has a prime duty to maintain professional competency in terms of knowledge and ability of new medicine, device and technology as and when available as a health information advance. Pharmacist also should have competency in up gradation of knowledge in old medicine, device and technology etc. They have responsibility to maintain personal, physical and mental health to serve patient. Pharmacist must participate in research, survey or project work associated with health care system which are carried out in ethical and scientific manner and approved by appropriate agency in the benefit of country or public at large. Before participating in research pharmacist should obtain informed consent of the patients whose data will be used in such research work without disclosing identity of patient. Pharmacist must inform patient about aim, objective, purpose, resource of funding, harm and benefit, nature of participation of project. It should be informed to the patient that information of participant will be kept confidential and not disclosed without his/her consent or permission. Pharmacist should engage in education of students, inter and residential education including multidisciplinary and collaborative training and experience. Pharmacist should participate in continuous education and continuous evaluation programs. He should develop, promote, and participate in quality improvement and quality assurance programs. The advanced knowledge acquired by him should be made available for patients and colleagues and society.

Value of Colleagues

Pharmacist must respect the value and ability of colleagues and other health professionals. The knowledge of professional colleagues and other health care professional differs. The other professionals might be specialized in other areas of science where pharmacist is not. This difference in specialization and knowledge pharmacist should respect. When found appropriate pharmacist should ask patient or refer patient for consultation of colleagues or other health care professional. Pharmacist should act with honesty and integrity in all professional relationship and fulfill responsibilities as per code of ethics. He should uphold spirit of code of ethics.

Services

Pharmacist should provide services and he should serve for patient, individual, community and for social need. The prime obligation of pharmacist is service to patient. However obligation of pharmacist might be extended beyond individual patients to the health of community and society. In this condition pharmacist should decide the priority and act accordingly. Pharmacists are committed to protecting and promoting well-being of patient and community. Pharmacist should practice in scope of his education, training and competency. He is well aware of about limitations of knowledge and expertise in health care management and should refer the patient as and when found necessary and appropriate. Pharmacist should adhere to national and state laws, legislation standards and policies. Pharmacist should maintain adequate resources to deliver services as per standards.

Distribution of Health Resource

A pharmacist should seek justice in distribution of health resources in fair manner. When pharmacist is allocated a responsibility of distribution of health resources, the distribution of such resources should be done fair, equitable and in balances manner to fulfill the need of patient and society. Pharmacist should ensure not to engage in discrimination based on age, gender, race, cultural difference, national origin, religion, lifestyle, presence of disability, socio-economic status or on the basis of prescriber.

Professional and Situational Ethics

The profession of pharmacist is governed by code of ethics. The constitution of Pharmacy Council of India has given us legal binding through Drugs and Cosmetics Act. Moreover, India is a country having diversified religions living together. As a professional pharmacist he cannot void the legal binding of Drugs and Cosmetics Act. As a responsible pharmacist he has to obey the code of ethics and as a responsible citizen of India he has to respect each civilian and religion. In such complex situations there might be conflicts in professional and situational ethics. The pharmacist has to solve these conflicts using his knowledge, skill and attitude. Pharmacist should not violate legal requirement, follow the code of ethics and respect the religion during solving such problem. The example of such conflict are quoted below *(These cases are presented as an example and - not happenned or experienced by any pharmacist at any place. This is only imagination).*

Case No. 1: Various complaints were received by office of food and drug administration that a registered pharmacist working in a drug store refusing to fill the authentic prescription of oral contraceptive tablet when he realizes that the tablets were used as a "morning-after therapy". When reason was asked to him about his act, he answered that "his religion beliefs do not condone abortion". As an Indian citizen he has right to keep his religious belief, but as a registered pharmacist he cannot refuse to fill the prescription.

Case No. 2: Doctors prescribe a powerful tranquilizer to a well educated patient. But telephonically he directed to the pharmacist that "dispense the powerful tranquilizer but label it as mild sedative. It is part of his therapeutics because patient is frightened by idea of taking tranquilizers. The drug prescribed is only the effective therapy for his condition". As per State Pharmacy Council law, mislabeling is strongly prohibited but as per code of ethics, pharmacist should do the things in the interest of patients well being.

In case no. 1 the question is that does the pharmacist working ethically in particular situation? Does the pharmacist affirm ethical stand? Does pharmacist has basic human rights and duties? What is code of ethics for pharmacist? In case no.2 the question is that what will happen to the State Council law about mislabeling? What are the rights of physician during prescribing and giving treatment to the patients? Does issue about patient's right for his betterment allow this?

Ethical dilemma occurs when there is disagreement on certain point or even between pharmacist and patient, pharmacist and physician. The dilemma between pharmacist and physician can be resolved because both of them has common point of interest that is well being of patient. The dilemma is due to difference between ethical behavior, application of ethical behavior, difference in values, sense of justice, fairness. Physicians were most often affected by dilemma. However in cascade reaction pharmacists are also affected as they also come in direct contact with patients. The action of pharmacists were affected due to legal liability, real and perceived. Pharmacist tries for maximum patients care and minimum legal liability. The inter-collegial relation may become strained under such dilemma condition.

Pharmacist and other members of health care management team regularly face such kind of dilemma regarding balancing between legal rights of patients and their autonomy, paternalistic attempt. Pharmacist sees the best interest of patient without attempting the legal consequences. All the members in health care management chain should utilize their capabilities of decision making using various theories and concepts to solve ethical dilemmas that they face in practice. These value based decisions are the landmark of profession and values essence of pharmacy practice such as compassion, faithfulness, altruism, justice and equality.

Code of Conduct

Profession

The behaviors of pharmacist towards his profession include proud, responsibility and competency. Moral obligations for profession are must rather than legal. There are no legal obligations regarding profession, but pharmacist must have moral obligations towards his/her profession.

- **Proud:** When student select pharmacy as a profession it becomes his/her integral part of profession. The afterall every member of pharmacist contribute for profession on his own way for the betterment of profession. Being a student of pharmacy or pharmacy professional we should develop our mental, physical and social ability to be proud of pharmacy profession. This does not give an immediate outcome but help in later period for professional development. The personal gain will be professional satisfaction and happy professional practice.
- **Responsibility:** Pharmacist is a member of one of the noble profession and hence voluntarily he should accept the professional responsibilities. Pharmacist should accept all the responsibilities of professional activities undertaken by himself or under his supervision. Pharmacist has heavy responsibility of health care of patients. One might found it difficult to handle multiple responsibilities. Pharmacist should learn to accept and execute these responsibilities by appropriate decision making. The mistakes encounter during professional life of pharmacist must be accepted honestly, it must be overcome immediately and learned not to repeat the same in future.
- **Competency:** Pharmacist come across with different type of patients at various instances like dispensing, counseling, ward round etc. Various questions may be raised in front of him by patients, physicians, colleagues, fellow pharmacist etc. Pharmacist has to answer these queries and questions and to do so he must have competency. The competent pharmacist will become successful in his professional career and will be satisfied. Competency of pharmacist is central point in his career development. Hence pharmacist has prime responsibility to maintain his competency by continuous

education, attending seminars and conferences, updating knowledge etc.

Patients

Patient is key person in health care management system. Everything in health care management circle rotates around patient. Every member of health care management team works for the benefit of patient. Pharmacist is also at prime location in health care management team. His relation with patient governed by various factors which include his attitude, relationship, goodness, autonomy and dignity towards patients.

- **Attitude:** Pharmacy, medical and nursing profession provides services to the patients. The service given by these professionals is beyond the boundaries of religion, caste, category, gender etc. hence it is believed that service to sick and ill is service to God. The pharmacist must have caring attitude towards patients so that it's a service to God. Caring attitude in the pharmacist will develop with expression of sense of belonging and love. It should have only attitude and language will not be a barrier. This attitude should be like the caring attitude of mother towards her child or priest give care to his devotees. The caring attitude of pharmacist with patient should be with concern and empathy. Pharmacist should understand the situation of patient and feeling for him without getting involved emotionally in it and becoming upset.
- **Relationship:** The code of ethics adopted by American Pharmacist Association (APhA) in 1994 defines relationship between pharmacist and patient. Pharmacist should respect these relations with moral obligation. The relationship of pharmacist with patient should be covenant. Covenantal relationship is a gift of trust. In return of this gift pharmacist provides optimum benefit to the patient.
- **Goodness:** As a center for professional practice pharmacist should provide all good in the patients caring in sympathetic and confidential manner. This is for well being of patient. Pharmacist must look in to the needs of the patient, science of illness, need as per therapeutics and his authorities before doing goodness.

- **Autonomy and dignity:** The philosophy of health care management is communication with patients regarding his illness and intended therapy. It is legal right of patient to know about his illness, disease, abnormality etc., and intended therapy for it. Pharmacist should respect this autonomy of patient with dignity. He should communicate the patient about illness, medicine, its use and other associated aspects which are in his purview. The patient should be treated with courtesy, autonomy and dignity during communication and therapy. Pharmacist should ensure that with maintaining autonomy and dignity, patient should get all the information he/she want to seek.

Himself

For the self confidence, dignity and job satisfaction factors that contributes pharmacist himself also play important role in professional life. Control of emotional and mental thoughts, self discipline, honesty and integrity, courage, personal appearance, mental, emotional health status are important contributors of successful pharmacy professional life. Over expectation, non-satisfaction from job may land the pharmacist in the condition of frustration and this ultimately affects his performance in professional life.

- **Emotional and mental thoughts:** While at work, professional pharmacist should control his emotional and mental thoughts. This ability indicates his stable and balanced personality and mental condition. This balanced and stable mental condition is must for safe handling of prescription and during counseling of patients. Pharmacist should show the sensitivity toward patient but should not get involve in mental and emotional status of patient. Pharmacist has to work with variety of patients including depressed or having psychiatric illness. The mode of operation towards this varying patients should be balanced and as per need of patient. In all the variable circumstances pharmacist should behave in balanced manner. If pharmacist is affected by mental or emotional thoughts he will fail in his professional activity and will fail in rendering the services to the patient. He will lose his dignity and graciousness.

- **Discipline:** It is always expected from pharmacist to work without rest. Like other health care professionals he works in different situations and much is expected from him by patients. During their academic, education and training pharmacists are exposed to various opportunities where they will have a feel of discipline in life. However to maintain the consistency in performance pharmacist requires continuous training and efforts to adapt to the situations. The discipline is set by authorities to aim the quality services for patients. The professional pharmacist should understand the purpose of discipline and avoid deviation from their set point. The purpose of discipline is to make pharmacy services more professional and acceptable to the patient and not to impose rules and regulation on them in order to punish. With age, experience and understanding pharmacist become self disciplined and learned the importance of punctuality. Discipline and punctual pharmacist will be respected by all. Pharmacist must use dress code, identity card and should be physically present in working time.
- **Honesty and integrity:** Pharmacist can have long pharmacy practice career with association of honesty and integrity. He should have honesty and integrity in all professional relationships. It is important to provide good services to the patients. The good services can only be provided if pharmacist is honest and integrated with his services. Pharmacist should always be truthful, sincere and fair in his professional life when dealing with patients and other customers. Punctual and accurate at work, fair in dealing with patients, their relatives and friends, keeping promises, using resources in fair way, respecting other individuals and their belongings are the other characteristics of being honest pharmacist and integrated in professional life.
- **Courage:** Courage means brave or not to afraid of. Pharmacist requires courage in his professional life. Courage is quality in practice and may not be recognized always. Knowledge gives power to career and it is essential for courage. Pharmacist should not be afraid to any adverse situation encountered during his professional life. A commitment in professional life along with confidence, knowledge and capabilities helps in getting courage. Starting pharmacy education in 1932 at

Banaras Hindu University by M. L. Schroff, starting clinical pharmacy practice by American Pharmacist in 1950 and 1970, starting hospital pharmacy course at Delhi University in 1982 are some of the examples of courage of the pharmacist who brought revolution. Courage is required to accept the mistakes and to follow the truth.

- **Appearance:** It is always saying that first impression is always last impression and long lasting impression. In daily professional working pharmacists come across with different patients, physicians, fellow pharmacists and individuals. It is creating impression of him. His appearance will have a strong impact on impression. Pharmacist might not have a second opportunity to show impression again. A clean neat, simple, pleasant, official appearance should be preferred; it provides peace of mind with in working hours. Having casual wearing during professional life indicate that you are not serious enough during professional hours, where you must be serious enough during dealing with patients. Pharmacist must wear white overcoat during his professional working hours whether in community pharmacy, hospital or counseling centre. Wearing identity card gives a professional look to pharmacist. This professional look of pharmacist gives impact in society that he is the person who cares for your life and illness. Some hospitals, organizations and pharmacy departments have their own dress code and code of ethics of dressing.
- **Health:** The professional performance of pharmacist is influenced by physical, mental and spiritual health. Well maintained health status is must for pleasant, dynamic and confident act. Physical health condition of pharmacist (in all aspects) will help him to have good posture and work without fatigues during monotonous working hours. Mental health conditions empower him to combat and manage emotional and stressful situations. Pharmacist must know and well understand the religious belief of patients and customer in order to meet their needs and demands. Religions framework affect the behavior and emotional status of individuals differently. He should work in frame work of religions belief. Spiritual health of pharmacist will play a very important role in this situation.

Society

Society is a place where from the stake holders of health care system are coming. It is also a part where we all stay and spent our life. The attitude and behaviors of pharmacist towards this -stake holder should be in an aim and objective of providing services, in an attempt to have a balanced life style, with social and professional adjustment, with learning attitude, problem solving capabilities and participation in professional organization and associations.

- **Service:** Providing services to the individual patients is primary obligation of pharmacist. Pharmacist may extend his services to the need of community and society. Pharmacist first must understand the primary obligations and then participate in the community health programs. His participation in such community programs should not affect the primary services to the patients. Providing cost effective medicine to the needy patients (by using a generic substituent) is the best example of professional obligation. Dispensing of prescription accurately, with minimal waiting time, giving accurate and authentic information about medicine within framework of authorities are also the professional obligations of the pharmacist towards patient and society.
- **Balanced life style:** Pharmacist should have a balanced life style. Only engagement in professional life and complain about not having time for other activity is dangerous situation and such condition should be avoided. The balanced life style includes participation in various activities along with professional activities like social programs, religious activities, cultural events including recreation and domestic activities. Professional pharmacist has responsibility to develop interest and relationship in all areas and make life style well balanced. Pharmacist must show interest and should participate in activities of community and society. Participation in religious activity helps him to feel more fulfilled as a person. Development of good friends circle helps him to achieve excellence in professional life. Recreation activity will help pharmacist in relieving work tensions due to professional or other duty. The balanced life style make pharmacist loyal, dependable, gentle, resourceful and cooperative. Pharmacist will easily understand the need of other and promote other to have balanced life styles alike him.

- **Professional adjustments:** For a person to be happy, adjustment and acceptability is must in the life. Adjustability should not be compromised with honesty, dignity, loyalty, faithfulness and truth in the profession. The adjustment means adjusting to the changing scenario of pharmacy practice services and technology updating. The success of professional pharmacist depends on how much he will adjust to fit the new systems and situation. It also depends on willingness to accept the adjustment. The changes should be accepted willingly. Forceful adjustment will decline the performance of pharmacist and may leads to situation of frustration. Pharmacist has to adopt and adjust the change in environment. Development of friendship, cordial relation with others is important aspect of social adjustment. For the development of good professional relationships getting along with other is necessary.
- **Learning and continuous education:** We as a human being learn throughout our lifespan. We learn various things right from birth till death. Initially we to learn talk, walk at later stage. Learning involves doing complex things in professional manner. Learning is continuous and never ending process in life. Learning through experience is like trial and errors and it is a slow process. Participation in continuous education programs, content updating programs, seminars, conferences, library book reading etc. is systematic approach of learning process. According to Loretta E Heidgerken, learning is acquiring knowledge, skills, attitude, appreciation and ideas through mental activity. This results in modification of behaviors. Pharmacist should not believe that after acquiring degree of bachelor's, master's and doctoral his learning process is completed. It is continuous process and will never complete till end of life. To be a successful professional pharmacist must be student throughout his life. Pharmacist must imbibe this attitude in him. A pharmacist will be successful when he keeps the attitude of updating himself continuously by any means of media throughout his life span of career. Sharing the experiences is also one of the potential modes of learning. Professional pharmacist must share his experience with fellow pharmacist and other health care team members at suitable platform.

- **Problem solving capacity:** In the professional and personal life of pharmacist problem is integral part. Problem is usability to solve the difficulty for short period of time. For some period of time some person, certain event make the pharmacist troubled and unhappy and reduced ability to cope with simple difficulties in day to day activity. This unhappiness keeps the pharmacist away from normal professional activities and reduces his ability to solve the problem from any origin. Pharmacist requires greater efforts to perform simple tasks. At such moment pharmacist should recognize the problem, think about possible solution, analyze what - happened and what can happen- and select one of the best option as a solution or remedy for problem. If problem is resolved then the action is successful and it will add into your experience. If not second option should be tried and this will also add experience in your life.
- **Association with organization and associations:** Various associations and organizations are their which look after the professional development of the members and society at large. Such association and organization come in to existence with specific agenda. These association work for well being of the members of association and organize events for benefit of community. A professional pharmacist should join the suitable professional organization working in the field of his professional work and activity. Association of pharmacist with such organization will help him in different ways. It gives him feeling of belonging with associated professionals, various schemes gives security, get opportunity to develop leadership. Such organization will help their members in solving their common problems by providing platform for their say. Publication of journals helps them for content updating and sharing the experiences and ideas in their professional life. Such published journals also help them to inform about current events, knowledge in their field. Journal also provide opportunity to publish articles, write-up and to voice opinions of the members of association.

Other Health Professionals

Health care management system involves specialized individuals from various fields. Other health care professionals include surgeons and physicians from various specialization, nursing staff, counselor's administrative staff etc. The pharmacist should respect the values and abilities of each of them. Pharmacist should willingly accept the limitations of himself and each colleague. There are limitations for each individual in respect to knowledge, experience and practice. Pharmacist should ask for and give them consultancy for referring the patients. The limitation of knowledge, skill and attitude should not be used as weak point of individual but can become a strong point - with sharing the limited resources available with each - individual.

The concept and knowledge of each individual might be different. This difference might be their due to professional difference. The pharmacist must respect this difference and by knowing the limitation of pharmacy profession should act, behave and suggest the fellow professional. This difference in knowledge, beliefs and values they apply to the profession as per the code of ethics of each professional. Pharmacist should respect his own code of ethics and code of ethics of other profession also. In doing so as an individual pharmacist should follow moral, accountability.

Pharmacist's Oath

Hippocrates was regarded as father of western medicine. It is believed that pharmacist oath was first time written by Hippocrates in Greek language way back in late 5th century BC. The oath includes Hippocratic Corpus. Ludwig Edelstein proposed that oath was written by Pythagoreans. But his theory was questioned due to lack of evidence to support findings. Hippocratic Oath (orkos) was widely used in Greek medical text books. Hippocratic Oath is oldest binding document in history. It is written in antiquity. The principles of Hippocratic Oath are held sacred by doctors till date. The principles of Oath include treat sick to the best of physician's ability, preserve privacy of patients, and teach the secrets of medicine and its application to next generation. The American Medical Association's code of medical ethics (edition 1996) holds the basic principles of The Hippocrates Oath. It has remained in western country as expression of idea and conduct for the physician. Most of today's medical graduate students swear the modern version of Hippocrates Oath. The English translation of Hippocratic Oath adopted by Indian Medical Council (as published on their website) is as follows.

I swear by Apollo Physician, by Asclepius, by Health, by Heal-all, and by all the Gods and Goddesses, making them witnesses, that I will carry out, according to my ability and judgment, this oath and this indenture.

To regard my teacher in this art as equal to my parents; to make him partner in my livelihood, and when he is in need of money to share mine with him, to consider his offspring equal to my brothers; to teach them this art; if they require to learn it, without fee or indenture; and to impart precept, oral instruction, and all the other learning, to my sons, to the sons of my teacher, and to pupils who have signed the indenture and sworn obedience to the physicians' Law, but to none other. I will use treatment to help the sick according to my ability and judgment, but I will never use it to injure or wrong them. I will not give poison to anyone though asked to do so, nor will I suggest such a plan. Similarly I will not give a pessary to a woman to cause abortion. But in purity and in holiness, I will guard my life and my art. I will not use the knife on sufferers from stone, but I will give place to such as are craftsmen therein.

Into whatsoever houses I enter, I will do so to help the sick, keeping myself free from all intentional wrongdoing and harm, especially from fornication with woman or man, bond or free.

Whatsoever in the course of practice I see or hear (or even outside my practice in social intercourse) that ought never to be published abroad, I will not divulge, but will consider such things to be holy secrets.

Now if I keep this oath and break it not, may I enjoy honor, in my life and art, among all men for all time; but if I transgress and forswear myself, may the opposite befall me.

The Pharmacy Council of India in 1996 has adopted a pharmacist oath. The as it is version of the Oath is given here as below –

I swear by the code of ethics of Pharmacy Council of India in relation with the community and shall act as integral part of health care team.

I shall uphold the laws and standards governing my profession.

I shall strive to perfect and enlarge my knowledge to contribute to the advancement of pharmacy and public health.

I shall follow the system which I consider best for pharmaceutical care and counseling of patients.

I shall endeavour to discover and manufacture drugs of quality to alleviate sufferings of humanity.

I shall hold in confidence the knowledge gained about the patients in connection with my professional practice and never divulge unless compelled to do so by the law.

I shall as society with organization having their objectives for betterment of profession of pharmacy and make contribution to carry out the work of those organizations.

While I continue to keep this oath unviolated, may it be granted to me to enjoy life and the practice of pharmacy respected by all, at all times!

Should I trespass and violate this oath, may the reverse be my lot!

American Pharmaceutical Association, Academy of Students of Pharmacy/American Association of Colleges of Pharmacy Council of Deans (APhA-ASP/AACPCOD) has developed and adopted Oath in 1994.

At this time, I vow to devote my professional life to the service of all humankind through the profession of pharmacy. I will consider the welfare of humanity and relief of human suffering my primary concerns. I will apply my knowledge, experience and skills to the best of my ability to assure optimal drug therapy outcomes for the patients I serve.

I will do my best to keep abreast of developments and maintain professional competency in my profession of pharmacy. I will maintain the highest principles of moral, ethical and legal conduct. I will embrace and advocate change in the profession of pharmacy that improves patient care. I take these vows voluntarily with the full realization of the responsibility with which I am entrusted by the public.

References

5019 Code of ethics, College of Pharmacist of British Columbia, (July 2011) v2011.1.

American Society of Health System Pharmacists Inc (2013). Code of Ethics for Pharmacists. *In American Journal of Health-system Pharmacist* **52:** 2131.

Arden Barry, Nicole Bruchet, Jennifer Kendrick, Leanne Kwan, Sam Louie (2009). Is It Ethical for Health Care Organizations to Charge Institutions for Experiential Rotations?. *CJHP* **62(4):** 331-334.

Buchholz, Rogene A. and Rosenthal, Sandra B (1998). Business Ethics, Englewood Cliffs NJ.

Cicely Roche, Felicity Kelliher (2009). Exploring the Patient Consent Process in Community Pharmacy Practice, *Journal of Business Ethics* **86:** 91-99.

Code of Ethics for Pharmacist (1995). *Am J Health-Syst Pharm* **52:** 2131.

Code of Ethics for Pharmacist 2011, Pharmaceutical Society of Australia, www.psa.org.au.

Code of Ethics for Pharmacist, American Pharmacist Association (APhA), www.pharmacist.com.

Code of Ethics for Pharmacists and Pharmacy Technicians, Royal Pharmaceutical Society of Great Britain, www. rpsgb.org.

Farnell, Lewis R (2004). The famous Hippocratean oath may not be an authentic deliverance of the great master, but is an ancient formula current in his school, "Chapter 10". Greek Hero Cults and Ideas of Immortality. Kessinger Publishing. ISBN 978-1-4179-2134-8, pp. 234–279.

Goodpaster, Kenneth E (1992). Business Ethics, in L.C. & C.B. Becker, eds., Encyclopedia of Ethics, New York, 111-115.

http://en.wikipedia.org

Johannes Brinkmann (2002). Business Ethics and Intercultural Communication. Exploring the overlap between two academic fields, Intercultural Communication. http://www.immi.se/intercultural.

K.G. Ravikumar, B.D. Miglani (2009). A Textbook of Pharmacy Practice, 1st edition, Career Publications.

Remington (2005). The Science &Practice of Pharmacy, 21st ed., Lippincott Williams & Wilkins.

Robert A. Buerki, Louis D. Vottero (2002). Ethical Responsibility in Pharmacy Practice, American Institute of the History of Pharmacy, Madison, Wisconsin, Second edition, ISBN 0-931292-37-9.

Robert A. Buerki, Louis D. Vottero (2008). Foundations of Ethical Pharmacy Practice, American Institute of the History of Pharmacy Madison, Wisconsin, ISBN 978-0-931292-42-2.

Temkin, Owsei (2001). On Second Thought and Other Essays in the History of Medicine and Science, Johns Hopkins University, ISBN 978-0-8018-6774-3.

The Hippocratic Oath: Text, translation and interpretation By Ludwig Edelstein (1943), ISBN 978-0-8018-0184-6, Page 56.

The Hippocratic Oath: Text. Translation and Interpretation, by Ludwig Edelstein, Supplements to the Bulletin of the History of Medicine, (1943), no. 1.

Translation from the Greek by Ludwig Edelstein. From *The Hippocratic Oath: Text, Translation, and Interpretation*, by Ludwig Edelstein. Baltimore: Johns Hopkins Press, 1943 from The hippocrate oath today.html.

Website of Indian medical Association, http://www.ima-india.org

Werner Lowenthal (1988). Ethical dilemmas in pharmacy. *Journal of medical ethics* **14:** 31-34.

Index

A

B

C

I

O

P

Q

R

www.ingramcontent.com/pod-product-compliance
Ingram Content Group UK Ltd.
Pitfield, Milton Keynes, MK11 3LW, UK
UKHW021325190726
13845UKWH00003B/42